# A Diary of Walter's
# Backseat Driver

# A Diary of Walter's Backseat Driver

Janet Boyle

**VANTAGE PRESS**
New York

Each individual should seek the advice of his or her own physician before starting any new medical program. The opinions and instructions expressed herein are solely those of the author.

FIRST EDITION

Published by Vantage Press, Inc.
419 Park Ave. South, New York, NY 10016

Manufactured in the United States of America
ISBN: 978-0-533-15632-0

Library of Congress Catalog Card No.: 2006908529

0 9 8 7 6 5 4 3 2 1

I lovingly dedicate this book to three very special individuals. To Walter, a man whose life experiences touched me and many others through very special, personal and unique ways as he journeyed along his road through life. He gave me the inspiration to find the strength and courage within myself to recognize the important things at a time when his own life was nearing its close. His experiences gave me the inspiration to write. It was a story which began with his own struggle, but which inevitably taught me some very valuable lessons along the way. Walter showed me how a single individual, regardless of what stage of life they were in, still had the power to touch other people and help them along their own personal journeys.

To Maggie, a soul I had never known or even met. She provided me with a sense of spiritual understanding and friendship as I struggled along this journey during a time in which I felt I was very much alone. I often thought about this wonderful and dedicated woman many times over the years and I drew on her own story as I struggled through the difficult times as my life's story was continuing. I wished I had known Maggie. I would have told her that her own story had special meaning for me and it had changed my life.

And to Robert, a man who encouraged me and listened with interest as I would recount how the family made its way through many difficult challenges as we cared for Walter. Robert helped me to recognize the humor within ourselves as I described how we, as loving children, were suddenly thrust into the role of well-meaning yet highly unqualified caregivers almost overnight. He related to our loving yet sometimes unconventional methods of finding solutions to even the smallest of challenges. As the son of an aging parent himself, he believed I had a story worth telling. He believed that my story may help someone else, and he encouraged me to write it down.

# Contents

# Introduction

Walter was a kind and gentle soul. It was his destiny to experience the disease known as Alzheimer's as he finished his journey through life. "Alzheimer's" was a word we all heard over the years and often used it glibly ourselves when we couldn't find our keys or remember a phone number. There was no warning of the silent events methodically taking place within our close knit family . . . or maybe there was. Looking back on the events now, I think lovingly of Walter progressing gently and quietly through each stage as if everything were in control, untouched and as it should be, while his family and friends spiraled out of control at times and buzzed around in a frustrated, panicked frenzy in search of normalcy.

We became his back seat drivers on his road of life, guiding his every move and at frustrating times, barking out direction. His response was always the same, a gentle smile and a word of thanks. This is our diary as we dealt with fear, grief, stress, denial and finally acceptance as we watched our loved one slip away from our world of understanding. Yet the power of love and humor became our story as we discovered that his journey was really our own journey as well. He touched each of us as we were learning our own individual and very personal life's lessons along the way. This self-discovery was his special gift to each one of us, as Walter was a kind and gentle soul.

# I

# "Maggie"

I read the obituary, and then I read it again. There was no picture of her. I didn't know her and yet that bothered me. There should have been a picture. There was no mention of surviving children or a spouse, only her name and her brief life's story reduced down to two short paragraphs. Her name was Margaret and she was only fifty-two, hmmm . . . . not much older than me. The paper said she had given up her career with a marketing firm to care for her aging parents who were diagnosed with Alzheimer's Disease.

An interesting obituary which to me, confirmed all of the articles I had already read. It was often the children, who with the very best and loving intentions become care givers to their parents. They often overlook or become too involved in the rigorous daily routine to recognize the warning signs. They become in need of care themselves after a dramatic life style change which consisted of continuous stress, responsibility and worry. It was not uncommon for the aging parent to outlive the care giver, so the article said.

We would not become like Maggie. We would keep our heads on straight. After all, we are intelligent, rational and strong. Our family will become our network of strength. We are reading the right books, talking to doctors, and we are staying informed and involved. All we need is a well thought out plan . . . yah, that's it, a well organized, well thought out plan. The book says to develop a care-giving plan early in the process. That way, we can anticipate and plan ahead rather than reacting in a crisis situation. We will follow the practical advice outlined in the book. Practicality alone won't be enough. We will need emotional involvement to nurture our creativity, flexibility, a sense of humor and a "can-do" attitude, so the book said.

We will establish goals that will provide a supportive environment for our loved one. We will learn how to make his home a safe and secure environment. We will discover effective ways to manage difficult behavior. We will forge workable solutions to family conflicts about providing care for Dad. We will develop ways to protect ourselves from "care giver burnout." We will be able to pull Dad through this with strength, patience, control and steadfast perseverance until the end. We are real troupers and this is just another challenge. After all, how hard could it be anyway? No . . . no way . . . we would not become like Maggie.

Maggie became that one special soul who I would think of many times over the following years. As each day brought unexpected challenges and emotions which roller-coasted up and down without warning, I began to think of ourselves as that fellow in the circus. He's the one who has all the spinning plates in the air up on sticks, running frantically from one to the other, giving a spin to the plate that needed it most and then running to the next, and so on. How long could we keep up the flurry of having to keep all these plates in the air at the same time, revisiting each plate time after time and then running to the next?

With one false move, one skip in the routine or one momentary distraction and the whole thing will most likely come crashing down. What about that well organized, well thought out plan? What happened to that strength, that patience, control and steadfast perseverance? Where the hell was a friend like Maggie when you needed her? She would certainly understand when no one else possibly could.

# II

# The Original Backseat Driver

I first met Walter more than twenty years ago. I remember that day very well. He first impressed me as a very strong and handsome man, quiet and polite. He carried with him a great presence which I grew to understand and respect over the years. He had a gentle quality. I always said that he was the only person I knew who never had anything bad to say about another human being. He had a charming and subtle wit, and I often found myself laughing out loud at his jokes even when no one else seemed to get them. He would give me that quick glance with a twinkle in his eye and a little smile on his lips as I laughed.

It was many little private moments like that which we shared over the years which made my role as his daughter-in-law a very special one to me. Walter had three sons but no daughters, and I seemed to find my way to that very special place in his heart, and he in mine. I can honestly say that I learned a lot from that man by the kind and gentle way he treated people. I watched and listened, and learned to become a better person through his example. I always felt that if he ever needed me, I would be there for him and help pull him through whatever the situation, no questions asked, as I saw him do the same for many people in need over the years.

The signs were all there and yet we couldn't see the forest through the trees as they say. Oddly enough, it was a sign, an actual old wooden sign which was our first sign that something was wrong. It all started simply, a non-event. It seemed that Dad was worried about his sign and sign post which were near the highway that needed a little care and repainting. This was several years before Mom died, I think. The commercial sign was on Dad's property. It was actually an advertisement for his tenant's small restaurant business, but Dad always took pride in his property and was meticulous in making sure it looked nice and was well maintained.

Dad had his own tools of course, but on this particular day, David, Walter's oldest son, let Dad use his scraper, hammer and wire brush, as Dad's were old and rusty. David asked Dad to make sure he took care of them as David was very particular when it came to taking care of his tools. A few days later, David asked Dad if he was done using the tools, and Dad replied, "What tools are those?" He had no recollection of the tools or even fixing and repainting the sign. Dad was confused and very quiet. He just shook his head, as he could not recall a thing.

David explained to Dad how he had lent the tools to him several days before and even took him to see the repaired and freshly painted sign. Dad just stood there confused, now wondering who had painted his sign. Then Dad said he may have put some tools away in the garage. David searched the garage and yard and no tools were to be found. It was a puzzle, but the incident was kind of forgotten. Three years later, a company was hired to bring in a backhoe to even out some bumps and gullies on the property.

Mom and Dad's old compost pile was being leveled and the driver stopped as he saw some metal objects turning up in the dirt. The driver was puzzled and excited to see that the items were tools. David came over for a look. There they were, his once beautifully cared for tools, now rusted and ruined. Dad probably had put them in a bucket, and then used the same bucket to pick up grass clippings, and somehow the whole thing became compost. Well, you know . . . these things happen.

That following spring, David was helping Walter with the annual tilling of his garden. Like they had done for many years, they made long, evenly spaced corn rows, and mounds or hills for the squash plants. Dad, who had done this same routine for at least sixty-five years of his life, suddenly could not figure it out. The corn was normally planted with two or three seeds together, move down the row a foot and repeat. David noticed he was having trouble counting, and was just kind of randomly placing handfuls of seeds here, there and everywhere.

The same thing occurred when it came time to plant the squash. Squash was to be planted in hills with about four or five seeds per hill. Dad just couldn't count. Some hills had a handful of seeds, some hills had none. In the end, he forgot or just lost track of where he was and which hills had what. David had to dig up all of the hills see where he left off, and to straighten out the ones which were overseeded. Well, you know . . . these things happen.

During those next few years, David and his brothers became even more concerned. David was helping Walter for a couple of weeks during the summer. They were painting Dad's commercial building for the tenants. It was during this time that David would give Dad a small task, like painting the trim on a certain window frame. Dad would be on one side of the building, and David would be on the other, preparing the walls and mixing the paint. David would set Walter up with his paint and brush in front of the window where he was to paint, and then give him simple directions. David would return to his part of the building to resume work.

Every few minutes, Dad would appear back in front of David, confused and repeatedly asking for instruction on what he was supposed to be doing. David would explain and Dad would go back to his task. Moments later he would reappear, confused, and asking where the paint was. Back again . . . this time he did not know what he did with his brush. This is when David really first suspected there was a serious problem. Up until this time, little incidents were just brushed off. They were only happening once every couple of months or so, so there was no sense getting all upset and overreacting, right? You know . . . these things happen.

We were now all starting to take notice and we began to make mental notes on some of Dad's unusual behavior. No one really wanted to talk about anything they were noticing. It would be disrespectful after all, to say or imply bad things about Dad out loud. One day we received a call from a worried neighbor. Dad had decided to repaint his mailbox at the end of his driveway. The neighbor watched and had noticed Walter's confusion with the whole process of the paint can, repeating the process of opening the can, closing the can, opening the can, closing the can. Worst of all, Dad thought nothing of standing in the road while he was doing this. Cars were beeping, swerving and the drivers were making hand gestures. Dad would just smile and wave at them. He would continue on with his task as if he didn't have a care in the world, whistling as he painted.

One fine day, we noticed that all of the trash bins and wastepaper baskets in the whole house were missing. The one under the kitchen sink, the ones in all the bathrooms and bedrooms, wastepaper baskets in various other rooms . . . all missing. We searched the house, we searched the garage. We searched outside. We made our way across the yard, across the road, across the parking lot and all the way to the far end of Dad's commercial property. There was a dumpster there. It was a crazy idea, but we decided to have a look anyway. We opened the dumpster lid to find every last missing garbage can and wastepaper basket, maybe five or six in all. He had thrown them all entirely away.

Okay . . . so what kind of excuse shall we make up this time. First of all, it was really not so bad, now was it? No real crime had been committed. After all, he may have been a little confused, but he knew to throw the garbage away and so he did. That part was good. Besides, we asked Dad about it and he had no idea who would have done such a thing. Maybe it was someone else. Yah . . . that's it. Some horrible and twisted person must have broken into the house, completely bypassing the silver and the family jewels, just to make off with the dust bins. Then, overcome by guilt at their dastardly crime, disposed of the evidence.

David was having the property re-paved for Dad. Men and large equipment arrived one morning to begin the job. Walter was not just a nuisance, he was becoming a hazard and was ruffling the feathers of the workers. David had to repeatedly tell him to stand back, to get out of the way and things like that. He would walk out behind the heavy equipment, and the drivers simply could not see him. Walter did not respond to the "beep . . . .beep . . . beep" backup warning sounds these large trucks made.

Walter had lost all concept of danger. This was a man who had spent many years of his life working for a drilling and blasting company. He and his team worked with explosives. Safety was the highest priority in that line of work. He never took chances. Now he had to be escorted to his home and was directed to sit in his chair and commanded not to move.

Walter's driving skills had become a danger to himself and to everyone else on the road. Although we had begun to notice signs several years ago, it seems we began the process of "lowering the bar" as each small incident occurred.

This pattern of accepting and justifying each small occurrence as "not so bad" slowly changed our judgment as to what was normal. It seems that his wife, Anne, was doing a full-time job of cleverly concealing the magnitude of what was happening. She would carefully direct his every move while he was behind the wheel but even a short jaunt to the grocery store would become a challenge to fate.

Walter grew up in a small rural country town in Connecticut surrounded by farmland. One main beaten path made its way through the peaceful village years ago. Years later, the farmland became a maze of business development and that beaten path now a four-lane highway. It seems that Walter had this way of seeing his surroundings as they were maybe fifty years ago. Back then he might only have found an occasional vehicle passing by, and yet now he would continue to pull out across the four lanes without a care in the world. Horns would blow and chaos would unfold as oncoming traffic would dart for safety as the big black Buick found its way to one lane or another through bumper-to-bumper rush-hour traffic.

Angry faces and hand gestures did not change his gentle demeanor as he would merely smile and wave. We tried to convince Anne to take charge of the driving, yet she insisted that he was fine, becoming angry at times that we were perhaps insinuating that they were incapable. It was not until several years later, after Anne's death, that various friends would confide their hair-raising adventures as backseat drivers of the big black Buick. All agreed that it was Anne, barking out instructions, and usually just short of actually grabbing the wheel, who brought them all home to safety after these journeys.

Tales of driving the wrong way on highway ramps, crossing over medians and many, many close calls trickled back to us by way of reluctant friends. We were testing fate. This was serious business. There were innocent lives at stake. My inner self was becoming agitated, even angry. We have all got to start talking about this, openly and honestly. Looking back now, I shudder to think what could have happened. Denial and a deep-rooted respect for one's elders I suppose, made us participants in activity nothing short of criminal. Walter had another backseat driver as well. It must have been his Guardian Angel.

What seemed so painfully obvious to bystanders was not always so clear to those most close as we struggled with the emotional dilemma of taking away his independence. We reluctantly realized that we would have to step into the role of ''parent'' for the safety of everyone in his path. This was not an easy thing to do. Walter felt he was perfectly capable of driving his car and did not understand our concerns. Reasoning did not seem to work and he was very tricky. It seemed like cars keys were hidden all over that house in the most unusual places. We searched every nook and cranny to locate and confiscate them. The following day, as if by magic, another key would appear in his pocket.

We resorted to creating diversions and sneaking around, unhooking wires and removing the battery out from under the hood of the car when Dad wasn't looking. Eventually we won the battle. It was interesting to me how we as people were changing as well. We were nice, honest and caring people. We had begun having to use our Yankee ingenuity to always stay one step ahead of him. When that didn't seem to work we began polishing up our lying and sneaking skills. Funny how this worked so much better and we learned this all on our own. These skills were not to be found in the books.

It seemed that Anne was feverishly working to project normalcy at home as well, and she kept a vigilant eye on his every move before her death. As he would begin to stumble with the smallest of tasks, she was always ready to jump in and guide him with his daily routine, keeping up appearances and preserving his dignity. In the end, she was very reluctant to let go as she had become so proficient in protecting him. She was not ready to confide these dark secrets to her own children. One day near the end, we came through the door and found her crying quietly. She was sitting on the couch just looking at the wall, sniffing and holding her hankie. At first we thought it was because of her own struggle, having to face her own painful end. It wasn't that at all.

It seems that Walter had forgotten that they had two bathrooms in their house. Anne had looked out the window that day and saw him relieving himself in the yard. She was frantic and embarrassed. What if someone had seen him? What would they think? She dragged him back into the house, questioning him, yelling at him. He just didn't seem to know what he had just done, and he wasn't even aware of their indoor plumbing. She told us that this was not the first time something like this had happened. She still carefully guarded her biggest secret, the extent of Walter's progressing situation. I believe she felt we were not ready to pick up with her exhaustive role as secret caregiver. I don't think I ever gave much thought to or truly appreciated the depths of her love for him until that day.

With her death, things started unraveling quickly. Walter and Anne were always together. It was a teenage romance which lasted more than fifty years. They were never apart and her death left him tragically alone and confused. They were quite the pair. As we worked through our own grief of losing our mother, we struggled with watching the unbearable grief which he was suffering from the loss of his very best friend. It was during the most stressful of times, that we began to notice significant changes in Walter's behavior. We still seemed unaware, or unable to face the reality of the challenge we had in store for ourselves.

We were fortunate to have the kindness and support of Walter's physician to help us through the initial transition. As the trusted family doctor for many years, he was the one who with a gentle, professional yet heavy heart, had to deliver bad news to us on several occasions. We went to him to explain that behind closed doors, even the simplest of tasks were becoming difficult for Walter. Odd things were starting to take place. At one point, he could not remember the names of his three sons. He was retreating into his own world and was no longer interested in reading the paper or watching the news. His sense of humor never faltered, and he still made half-hearted attempts at telling jokes. We still continued to accept each little problem at home as "not so bad" and then we would lower that bar of acceptance just a little.

Dad was never one for visiting a doctor and felt that they only delivered bad news. At one point we felt that he may have had a small stroke of some kind and in for a visit he went. After many tests later, it was determined that he was very healthy for a man his age in all respects except for one. The tests for dementia indicated that he was most likely in the beginning stages of Alzheimer's Disease. Subtle changes were beginning to occur. Dad did not realize, but he had increasing forgetfulness, and made frequent attempts to cover it up. His efforts to cover up were valiant, but he was making mistakes. We noticed he had difficulty concentrating and had an inability to recall words. His sentences were becoming simpler.

Dad had problems with simple calculations and couldn't count money. He would study the bills in his pocket, but didn't seem to understand their value. I noticed he had trouble with any task which required fine motor ability, like buttoning his shirt or tying his shoes. At first I thought he may have needed new glasses when he struggled with getting the key in the lock, but I could see it was something more. He just couldn't deal with his simple daily life's tasks anymore. David was now managing his finances, tending to all of the household tasks, and helped Dad with maintaining his personal hygiene. The grim news became grimmer as we learned all we could about the disease and the different stages we would face with no happy ending.

I believed that when it came to taking care of a person with Alzheimer's, you needed to know as much as possible about the disease and how experts have learned to manage it. The disease progresses slowly, and changes take place gradually over time. People can live with the disease for about three to twenty-five years, although the average duration is about eight to ten years. I was busy reading and scouring the internet for information, remembering the old adage that "knowledge is power," and I believed that we could learn all we needed to stay in control and be one step ahead of the situation.

I typed the word "Alzheimer's" into my web search. There were 27,743,826 hits, articles and references referring to Alzheimer's. It was just so overwhelming. How does one begin this journey? I knew perfectly well that the journey had already begun. I needed to jump on board, and fast. Then one day I read a quote which rocked my knowledge boat a bit. A woman wrote "I always say . . . when you've met one person with Alzheimer's, you've only met one person with Alzheimer's." Every single case is unique. Knowledge is a great thing, but I haven't found an article or book yet to prepare me for Walter's most personal journey.

I digress back to Chapter I . . . We will be able to pull Dad through this with strength, patience, control and steadfast perseverance until the end. We are real troupers and this is just another challenge. After all, how hard could it be anyway? No . . . no way . . . we would not become like Maggie. I remembered that Anne looked up at me from her bed one night shortly before her death and she thanked me for all of my help. She studied me for a while, her eyes moving slowly across my face, and then she told me that she would help me one day. I smiled and bobbed my head, not really understanding. But now I am hoping that she will keep her promise.

# III

# Old Friends

There could be no more protected secrets and we needed help. Dad's confusion accelerated and I found it painfully apparent that friends and even some family members became distant in such a very short time. Even as we would voice our concerns to an occasional well-wisher, they would remark that Dad seemed "great," "perfectly fine." They said he could sit for hours and recall old times in great detail and never skip a beat. It seemed to me that he had this remarkable skill of picking up cues from bits of a conversation and could keep on talking as if all were well. I was secretly testing him myself. It was true. His memories of the old days were recounted in amazing detail, but when asked about incidents which occurred over the past few years, he struggled. When I would ask him about things which occurred that day, or even only an hour before, he seemed confused and unable to recount an event or series of events with any accuracy.

I became very aware of each word I spoke when asking him a question. I carefully chose my words. If I asked Dad, "Did you enjoy your lunch today?", he would enthusiastically respond that it was great and he ate every bite! One would think that all was well, that he remembered eating, that he remembered what he ate and that he liked it. If I instead asked, "Dad, what did you have for lunch today?", he would become silent and confused, not sure if he ate at all, and had no idea what he had eaten, much less if he enjoyed it or not even if he had just finished his meal ten minutes before. The response to this small bit of conversation had two entirely and dramatically different meanings. He was not "perfectly fine." He was proficient in chiming right along if a friend would say "Do you remember when we used to do this . . . or that?" Dad would enthusiastically agree to everything as if he recalled the events perfectly. I began to see how some could view his state as "perfectly fine," as it outwardly appeared that he knew just what they were talking about. If only they had asked him to recount something in a different way, then they would begin to understand.

I noticed that visits from old friends became fewer and far between. The old friends that insisted he was fine only served to make me angry. It was as if they were implying that we were making something out of nothing. Did they think we were just stirring up a scheme to get Dad out of our hair and into a home? Could they really not see what was happening, or was it just easier for them to look the other way? It was incredible to me. Perhaps we were not speaking loud enough.

Although Dad was living what would be perceived as an independent life, my husband David and myself would arrive each morning to assist with his shower, dressing and meal preparation. At noon time, David would break away from work to repeat the process. After work each day, I would meet David back at Dad's house for dinner preparation, cleanup and the bedtime coaching routine. Each day would bring more challenges as simple tasks became harder.

Dialing the phone and using the TV remote were small challenges for him that had now become impossible at times. We were faced with the constant fear of what was going to happen next. Winter was coming and we were afraid to leave him alone. He was living in the home he helped build more than fifty-five years ago, yet now he could not recall what doors in his hallway went where, or how to operate a light switch. Could he save himself if there were an emergency? We were not sure.

# IV

## Man's Best Friend . . . His Cat

To say that Dad was a lonely man did not even begin to describe what he must have been feeling inside. At times he would become quiet and retreat within himself. At other times, he would become visibly upset and openly grieve for Anne. I'm not sure which was worse. At first, we would take him for little visits to the cemetery, but only when he asked. We told him that we would take him, night or day, whenever he needed to go. I wanted to suck those words back in as quickly as they fell off of my lips. The man would have pitched a tent on top of Anne's grave to wait out his days if he thought he could get away with it. He asked to go all the time, and so we did.

His house was a shrine. Anne's photographs were everywhere. Flower arrangements which were sent to the house after her death, now sat dead in their vases all over the place. Sympathy cards were everywhere. He didn't want them touched. Her purse was still hanging on the doorknob. Her nightgown still hanging on the hook behind her door. I would make his bed every morning, and I sadly removed the carefully placed pillows from his bed. He would assemble pillows end to end to fill the spot where Anne had slept for all of those years beside him. I would make his bed and silently replace the pillows exactly as I had found them, carefully reconstructing the make-shift Mom.

17

After that very long first month, he stopped asking to go to the cemetery to visit her. We didn't ask why. We brought him there one last time, on her birthday, just after her stone arrived, but he didn't seem to realize why we were there. He didn't seem to know it was her birthday. We explained that we wanted to show him the stone. He read the engraved words with her name and dates sharply cut into the newly polished granite. Silently, he slowly ran his finger along each cut letter. He didn't say a word and he seemed too far away to really understand that she was gone. Maybe it was not him at all, maybe it was us who were too far away.

How I wished I could have come up with the right words to make things just a little better for him. I wished for just a little bit of wisdom to help ease his pain. There just had to be something I could do to make things better. I finally decided that it just might bring a little joy and purpose to Dad's life if he had a pet to care for. I had always felt that pets could be a great comfort for the elderly and the lonely and we needed to do something, anything to help Dad move on with his life. I needed to see Walter smile again. He was always an animal lover, especially fond of cats. At first this brilliant idea went over like a lead balloon and Dad was reluctant to have to care for a pet, but off we went to the animal rescue center anyway to find the perfect friend for Walter.

It was important that Dad's new friend chose us, and not the other way around. We walked the long stretch of wire cages and hoped for a sign. Most of the animals cowered to the rear of their cages, but we were drawn to one far away cage, where a small paw was reaching out to us. He was a beautiful little grey tiger striped animal with a playful twinkle in his eye. Within hours, Walter found joy with his new constant companion, his cat. Upon arrival with this new ball of fur, Dad agreed to "help us take care of our new cat for a while" as Walter always helped those who were in need of something. It didn't take long for Walter to forget that it was "our" cat and not his. I quietly smiled, somehow strangely proud of my newfound talent of trickery.

Dad loved his cat and his every topic of conversation would swiftly focus in on "Jake." Each night we would listen, as Dad would give an excited detailed accounting of his little boy's daily activities. It was not important to me if the detailed accounting was fact or fiction. What was important was that Dad had something new to focus on instead of grief. He was very happy to have this new responsibility and purpose. He spoke to Jake constantly in his soft, gentle and caring way.

Jake would listen with interest. Luck was on our side, as we were not landed with one of those aloof invisible type pets that only ingratiates themselves with the honor of their presence when they heard the sound of the can opener at meal time. Jake was a people-lover, always to be found on Dad's lap, or snoozing on the back of his chair. He was alertly on Walter's heels and followed Dad's every move. It was amusing to watch. It had to be a good thing to have Dad interacting with Jake all day instead of just sitting alone, silently in his chair as the long lonely hours ticked by.

I smiled as I thought of Mom once again. She would be happy . . . I think. We arrived one day to find at least a thousand little puncture holes, suspiciously resembling Jake's teeth marks, covering each and every inch of all six plastic place mats on the dining room table. Jake must have labored away for hours on that project. He also made himself right at home on her side of the bed. Did I also mention that Jake had turned Anne's favorite chairs, couch and other assorted furniture into his own personal "scratchy posts?" He was on his own little mission to shred every stick of furniture. That little boy had wreaked havoc on almost every inch of the place in no time. Still, you couldn't help but love him. He loved his Walter, and that was good enough for me.

Dad was sitting at the table having a snack, and there was Jake, sprawled out across the center of the table with one paw on Walter's plate. Jake thought nothing of snatching an occasional morsel right off of Dad's dish. I could picture Mom trying to break through from the great beyond, just to strangle Jake with her bare hands. This was one thing she never would have allowed. Nonetheless, Dad loved his little boy and took great care of Jake in his own way. In no time at all it was apparent that Jake was running the show. Sometimes Walter would ask about his other cat, although there was no other cat. That hardly seemed important. We would quietly and lovingly replace the breakfast cereal, or even the "Freetos" which Dad would place in Jake's bowl with actual cat food. Things were a little better for all of us since Jake took charge. Still, I had a nagging concern as things progressed.

There was going to come a day where Walter would need more care than we could handle. Maybe we could continue at home but maybe he would have to be moved to an assisted living facility. His little friend would be taken away from him and I just didn't want to put any type of sadness or separation into his already confused world. For now it was clear . . . Jake was the most important part of Dad's life. He was good company for Dad. I have always been an "everything in order," "stick to the plan" and "all ducks in a row" kind of person. It's a hard thing to let go of being anally organized your whole life and have to learn to live by a "take it day by day" approach. That sweet man is still teaching me things about myself. The days went by and for a little while anyway, things seemed better and Walter was much more cheerful. Jake needed Walter, and Walter needed Jake. Let's just keep smiling and press on.

# V

# The Home-Health-Aide Parade

In theory, the idea of the Home Health Aide seemed like the answer to our prayers. David was still checking in on Walter several times a day to keep things in order and rolling along. These pop-in visits sometimes lasted hours, depending on what David would find when he got there. This was now taking a toll on David's business. David has been self-employed as a welder for many years. He has had many loyal long time customers who were sympathetic to our family situation and even expressed admiration for the time David was spending taking care of his Dad. People patiently waited for their jobs to be completed, but even loyalty had its limits. Eventually David's business phone stopped ringing. I began worrying about paying the bills as now I was very concerned about the idea of being the sole provider. We were not going to make it on my salary.

We were really feeling the anxiety of leaving Dad alone at night after preparing his meal, cleaning up and getting him ready for bed. We would have to coerce him into eating and we even developed our own little routine of "tricks" to get him to eat. It was like negotiating with a small child who refused to eat his peas, only much sadder. I found myself planting my cheerleader happy face on as I pulled into his driveway after work each night. It was fake. I didn't want to be there and I didn't want to see any more signs of deterioration. Each night, the same thing . . . deep breath . . . . Then

I would walk through the door and bellow my big cheery "helloooo." Dad would call out the same, mimicking my sing-songy greeting.

Fear would race through me if I didn't hear him respond immediately. I would panic if I couldn't find him and I would timidly search the house and check the stairs to the basement, searching each room with caution until I could locate him. On the weekends, we would make several trips a day, delivering meals and making sure nothing dangerous was going on. We felt guilt and a growing fear each time we left. If we were not there, we were never far from the phone. We became home-bodies, always feeling as if something would go wrong if we dared to venture away from home . . . like to go the grocery store. We would race back home, relieved to find the phone was not ringing as we burst through the door. After several months we began to see that we were handling it, but not very well at all, and so we began the search for the perfect Home Health Aide to help us.

Being a Home Health Aide is a very admirable profession and it takes a very special type of person to take care of the elderly for a living. There are many, many reputable agencies to help families with caring for their loved ones. I had a job I loved many years ago when I was young. I decided that my sole purpose in life was to help people. I would help all those less fortunate around me. Gosh, I was a good person, a swell human being. I became an Operating Room Technician and served in the Medical Corps with the U.S. Navy. Every day was an exciting adventure for me back then. Later, after my enlistment was up, I found myself working for a short time with a private duty nurse's registry to care for the elderly in their homes. I thought it would be a very rewarding profession. I also worked as an aide for a local nursing home. I found it to be a tough job, both physically and emotionally, as you can't help but to become attached to those you care for.

I guess I saw the other ugly side too while working there which few people speak of. I saw the corporate reality and a system driven by the almighty buck. I saw neglect and my illusion that all health care givers were saintly was diminished. I made a career change early in life as I could never seem to separate my feelings, the professional from the personal I guess. I was feeling empty sadness while watching the elderly deteriorate and die almost every day. I never came across a happy ending in that line of work. I couldn't do it . . . I just couldn't do it anymore. I suppose I should have focused on the satisfaction of helping people who couldn't help themselves but I just didn't feel that way. I spent so much of my life working that I really needed to love my job.

We began the search for that unique and special person to care for our father. Of course they must have squeaky-clean credentials, impeccable work ethic, they must love their job and above all they must be kind. You know . . . someone just like me. We decided that we could keep up our regime during the week but to look for someone to care for him on the weekends. He didn't require any physical care per se. We were really looking for a companion to pick out his clothes, prepare a few light meals and to watch over him so he wouldn't wander.

The great thing about writing in a diary is that it becomes an outlet for one's true feelings. I once heard someone say "The truth is its own salve." When writing one's innermost feelings, one doesn't have to mince words just to be diplomatic. Let me restate that I have a huge admiration for the profession of home companion and care giver itself. Where would this world be without them? It's just that we didn't seem to have much luck in this area. Of the several aides we went through, they either didn't show up on time, or at all. One was skipping out early and billing us for hours they weren't even there. Walter wasn't eating as she would leave before he ate. We would find the food sitting there the next morning.

We decided that we should clarify the responsibilities, creating a detailed check-list of what we needed done by the aide on a daily basis. We all needed to be on the same page. I determined that we must not have communicated properly. My beautiful check-list was ignored. Sometimes I would arrive to an empty house and Dad's meal would be back in the refrigerator, sometimes it would be put back into the cold oven, but most times it was just sitting there on the counter. Things were left a mess and on one particular occasion, we popped in to check on things and Dad was nowhere to be found.

It was a hot summer day and the windows were all closed as the air conditioner was rumbling loudly away in the living room. We walked in and found our aide from hell stretched out on the sofa chatting on the phone with her friends. She didn't seem too concerned as we stood and waited for her to finish her conversation. We asked her where Dad was and what we got back was a blank stare. We searched for Dad and found him out in the backyard hovering over the pool, trying to stick tools into the pool filter from the looks of it. I knew if he got a shock or fell into the pool, she never would have heard him from inside the house over the noise of the air conditioner. If he had wandered off, he was only a short distance from the highway.

A million scenarios were going through my mind and the trust I was trying very hard to develop was gone. I wanted this to be the answer we were looking for, but it was not. We all wanted Dad to be able to stay in his own home for as long as possible. We thought about adult day-care but still would worry about what was going on in that house at night.

We both needed to continue working and we needed to find an answer which would give us peace of mind. David told me not to worry, that we could try someone else. Try someone else!!! I was enraged. This was our precious Walter we were talking about. We could not take chances. Now we would have to hire a second person to sit in the bushes to watch the aide who is watching Dad. But who can we hire to watch the bush sitter watching the aide who watches Dad? The Home Health Aide Parade ended swiftly. Back to original plan of doing it ourselves.

# VI

## Autumn

There is something special about the Fall. It was always my favorite time of the year and for the past twenty years or so, we had a special ritual of driving up to the Mohawk Trail to look at the leaves and to have pancakes at the Maple Sugar House with Mom and Dad. We would always stop on the way home to buy pumpkins, cider and chrysanthemums. This year was different. No more drives to Stockbridge for lunch or stopping on the side of the road so Mom could get out her clippers and swipe Bittersweet from "State-owned" land. No more clam bakes, family trips to Cape Cod, no more going as a family to all the little country fairs or just out to get an ice cream cone in the big black Buick.

I started seeing more of a rapid decline when it came to Walter doing simple tasks. He was having an especially confusing day and he was struggling again with the puzzle of the doors. The closet doors, the bathroom, bedroom, cellar and hallway doors. He couldn't figure out who put all those doors there. That's not so bad really, and we can just lower that bar a tad and pretend life is normal. We had taken all of the basic precautions outlined by the professionals. Major appliances were unplugged, dangerous chemicals and implements under lock and key. Who were we kidding anyway? We were still leaving him alone for many hours of the day and night.

A friend of ours told us a story she had read about a woman whose father had Alzheimer's. I was haunted by her story. There were just too many similarities. It seems that this man had begun to wander, and no matter what the woman did to prevent it, he always found a way out of the house. She too struggled for months with all of the challenges, fears and stress which go along with the discovery that your loved one is again missing. She finally resorted to finding her own creative solutions.

Apparently, after many failed attempts she came up with a brain storm. It was brilliant! It was simple, creative, unconventional and a wee bit sneaky. My kind of woman, whoever she was! In final desperation, she resorted to wall-papering the doors to match her walls, and she moved the door knobs and locks up a foot or so on all of the doors. That was all it took. The man no longer had the ability to rationalize the changes which were made and he never wandered again.

A story like that might be shocking, even offensive, or misconstrued as some form of abuse by someone who has not been touched in some way by this disease. I hope that people who are lucky enough not to be walking in the shoes of a care giver take care not to judge those of us who are. More and more people are abruptly confronted by just this same thing each day. My advice is this . . . be open to any and all possible solutions, conventional or otherwise which may help you to protect your loved-one. You may be amazed at what you can come up with when you put your mind to it. You will not find all of the answers you're looking for in the medical journals. I am personally saying a little prayer tonight with the hope that I shall not be wall papering any doors or moving any doorknobs in the near future. If I have to, I will, and my hat is off to those loving care givers out there who already have.

It was fall, and I just love fall. Halloween had always been a major production in my life. My own father always turned our old 1790s house into the town's favorite haunted house at Halloween and I would help him. Usually I would help plan and create elaborate new and improved macabre costumes in advance. For weeks, I'd be dreaming up spooky displays and special effects just to give the neighborhood kids a few hours of fun. Even as I got older, it was always the highlight of my October.

My enthusiasm had dwindled down to practically nothing this year and I had little energy left over to even stick a pumpkin on the front steps, but we had this idea that it would be fun for Walter to welcome the trick-or-treaters as he did every year. You know . . . carry on as usual. I arrived at his house with bags of candy in hand and a big giant smile on my face. My husband soon followed and we dumped the candy into two large festive Halloween bowls. I sat on the couch and watched silently as the events unfolded. David placed one bowl on each side of the inside front door and proceeded to do a practice run or "dress rehearsal" with his Dad to prepare him for the neighborhood kids.

David patiently coaxed his father with a pretend doorbell ring to have Walter to get up and go to the door, open the door, pick up a bowl of candy and offer it to the kids. This practice scene was replayed at least a dozen times. Each time his Dad would get up, but did not know where to go, did not know to pick up the candy, could not find the candy, and so it went. At one point David had me go outside and ring the bell. "Trick-or-treat," I said . . . still with that smile on my face. Walter did come to the door but could not think of what to do next and he didn't know why I was there. Even after repetitive coaxing and practicing, it became clear that this sequence of three small tasks was just too much for him. He would gently question what to do next and stood there puzzled. We decided it was best to click off the lights and lock the door. Walter went to bed. I cried all the way home. The next morning, we arrived to find Walter, completely fine and seemingly aware of everything around him.

# VII

# Jingle All the Way

The holidays are coming. I wonder how this is going to work. We are all beginning to really show the signs of stress, each in our own individual and very personal way. Me, I still have that planted smile on my face, prepared to dress up like Santa and rent a team of reindeer to drive across his front lawn if that's what it takes to have a jolly freaking Christmas. The old living day-by-day philosophy seems to be shifting to minute by minute. Every conversation is now about what to do with Dad. The endless routine, the endless dialog of hearing David instructing his Dad on proper showering and then sending him back in for a second time to do a better job. After Dad would dress himself, David would have him undress and replace the dirty layers of clothes with clean ones, as Dad often mistakenly put the dirty ones back on. Sometimes he would put the layers of dirty clothes over the clean, or vice-versa.

I would sit quietly at his dining room table, becoming irritated as David's tone would turn condescending at times. I listened as we performed the daily smoke detector test, quizzing Dad on what to do. I remember feeling my body become rigid as I held my breath. Every day, that pang of sadness as he wasn't answering quickly enough. I watched as Dad was given instruction on how to dial the phone. Large printed notes with our phone numbers hung everywhere on the walls. Reprogramming the phones for one touch quick dialing did not seem to work.

One night after arriving at our home, David and I started arguing about Dad. I don't even recall what started the whole thing. It must have been some small, insignificant dialog which exploded into a big mess. We were both tired from working all day and we were both worried about Dad. This was not particularly unusual as he consumed most of our energy these days. We were always worried, but that night we were unusually aggravated I guess. We tried to call and Dad did not answer the phone. We called and called again, by now in a panic wondering if he wandered off or fell in the pool. Maybe he was walking on the highway. Finally he answered and said he was fine, fine except for being confused when asked where he had been. He did not remember anything at all when it came to retelling the current series of events. He only knew he wanted to turn his TV off. David began the procedure of telling him how to locate the remote control. Back and forth . . . back and forth . . . and eventually he found it.

As David tried to explain which button to push, I could hear his voice rise and the frustration mounting in his voice as he repeated the instructions to his Dad over and over again. Walter was instead pushing the number buttons on the phone, and not the remote control, as I could hear the unmistakable beeping tones come through on our end. David just could not get him to understand to push the buttons on the remote, not the buttons on the phone. How could this be? He uses the remote many times during the day and never a problem. It was late and we were exhausted. David got dressed and made the nine mile drive back to Dad's to turn off the TV.

What seems to have added to the frustration was that the following day, Walter was back to his usual self, clicking the TV on and off like it's nobody's business, no problem. Were we dreaming up these problems? Were we just working ourselves into our own little frenzies? Let's just lower that bar of acceptance another inch because these small incidences are really not too bad. Then, a similar instance occurred a few days later. We could not make it to Dad's at the usual time to give him his breakfast and we didn't want him sitting there hungry. David called Walter and he began the process of instruction using very simple steps.

The process started with having Dad locate a bowl. Back and forth . . . back and forth . . . put down the phone . . . gone for a while . . . come back and hearing him ask again what exactly he is looking for . . . back and forth. The same endless procedure to locate a spoon. Again for the box of cereal, and forget about the milk, as he could not locate the refrigerator. At one point we could hear him opening and closing the microwave door but that's as close as we could get. One can not fully appreciate the frustration involved with directing the simplest of tasks, the tasks we all take for granted.

Many people have stated to us that it's just like training a child. How many times have I been told this and how many times have I said this is not true. They do not understand that a child can be trained through repeated guidance and eventually they learn. A child grows and learns. A parent can watch with pride as their child develops, conquers each task and begins to think and reason for himself. A growing child is a source of wonder and amazement. One can watch and only wonder about the amazing things the child will come to be through his life's experiences. This . . . is not that. We have not been able to train or retrain even the simplest of tasks. The instruction is not retained. It comes and goes at will and I think we are moving backward. There is no dreaming of tomorrow or a happy ending.

Okay, you can only play the cards that are dealt to you so let's say instead that the glass is half full. We already realize what we no longer have. What we have is still the innermost core of a wonderful human being. Sweet, gentle and always a word of thanks. I smile when I think of how Dad carries on at meal time. I will be the first to admit that I am not a decent cook. This is not a statement of modesty. I never was, nor ever will be, any good in this department. I was trying to fill some very big shoes here as Mom was the best at always creating delicious meals for him. It's really an art in itself I decided. Nontheless, I took it upon myself to "step up to the plate."

It didn't seem to matter what kind of concoction I would whip up for him. He was always full of thanks and praise, making those yum-yum noises as he ate, even if he was not quite sure what was presented to him at dinner time. He would not, under any circumstances, say or do anything to hurt my feelings. It was not in his nature to hurt anyone. Still, I felt in some small way that I was punishing him as I was quickly becoming famous in these parts as the "Queen of Cordon Blaaah." Then we heard about the most amazing thing . . . It was called Meals-on-Wheels. I came to the conclusion that Meals-on-Wheels was invented by Angels . . . or maybe God himself. At first skeptical, I soon began to appreciate how they helped so many people. I would arrive as usual to prepare a little gruel for his breakfast, but then each day, a friendly face would bring Dad his lunch, and his supper for us to heat up later.

The volunteers were all just amazing and each spent an extra moment to discuss the day's affairs with Dad. Occasionally they would bring a little extra secret treat for Jake. Dad really looked forward to their visits and enjoyed the food tremendously. I had spent my whole life focusing on my job and the daily rigors of my own life. While I was compassionate to the needs of the elderly, I never gave much thought to community service. I made a mental note that one day I would start giving back, and I would start by being one of these angels on wheels myself. The extra-added perk being that I would not have to actually cook anything. I could just be that happy face on the doorstep delivering those great meals. Imagine the joy of bringing the outside world in for some, or the joy of reaching out and maybe just making someone's day just a little bit better.

By now, David and his brother Raymond had made several visits to local assisted living facilities. We had become even more concerned with a harsh New England winter on its way. We really needed help but we were convinced that a move like this may just destroy Dad. We knew this move was coming but we couldn't seem to come to terms with the how, when and where of it actually happening. The hardest part for me comes with some of the things I have read about the progression of Alzheimer's Disease. I have fear of changes coming down the road. He seems to be progressing with what might be called textbook accuracy in all areas except for one.

Either God has shown divine mercy, or Anne has kept her promise to me. Many families have to deal with the heartbreak of personality changes. Usually the poor souls experience anger, suspicious and sometimes violent or accusative behavior as their condition deteriorates. We have been blessed with the most extraordinary gift. I always knew that this man had a true soul of kindness and a genuine good nature that fills him from the inside out. I can see this in him almost as a white light, a personality trait that goes so deep that it seems untouched by his other deterioration factors. Always, no matter what, his response is still the same, a gentle smile and a word of thanks. I think about him and I wonder what makes him different.

I believe that you are born, grow and are nurtured by those around you and you become who you are through each of life's experiences, both good and bad. Who you are changes through each of your life's experiences. I also believe you can sometimes personify traits and personality of who or what you want people to think you are. I believe that some people are very good at this, so good in fact that they may not be aware of it themselves through their whole life. I see these superficial traits as just the icing on the cake and I believe that with Alzheimer's, these traits are the first to go, as if you're being robbed of yourself, at first from the outside in.

The outer fluff or window dressing goes first, along with more of the mental and later physical capabilities. I think of this inner personality core as being the last to go, even if it can no longer be heard or reached. Not even Alzheimer's can rob a person of their soul. That is one thing I am sure of. It's just not possible. God would never allow that to happen. Hmmm . . . . Better ask me again this time next year. Perhaps I have this all wrong. For now, I'm just going to hold on to my belief. There are pressing issues at hand. I need to help Dad address his Christmas Cards.

A friend of mine called again to see if I wanted to go out to lunch, or maybe just go shopping with her. I politely refused, at least I hope I was polite. For God's sake, didn't these people realize that we had our hands full here? There wasn't time for such things. I did not live in their world anymore. We had something much more important going on here. When I did find a spare moment, I was learning valuable things from a book I was reading about caring for a loved one with Alzheimer's.

It taught me important things like "When moving your loved one away from their home, never say to people that you put Dad into a facility, say instead that you simply moved Dad." You should not say "facility" as it implies something clinical. "Moving Dad" is a much more polite , a more accepted phrase in society today. Oh yah . . . you are not supposed to say "patient" either, you are supposed to say "resident." Who writes this stuff, anyway? God forbid I should violate any rules of accepted phrases in society. And worse than that, I would hate to make anyone uncomfortable by saying something which sounds clinical.

# VIII
# Let There Be Light

I watch with amazement as I am starting to see some interesting survival techniques being developed here as Walter copes with new challenges. It's almost like he is digging deeper. He has to dig deeper as he loses the ability of maneuvering through regular everyday life problem solving. Some people may view it simply as erratic behavior, but if you stop for a moment and rethink, you can see the method to the madness. I believe it is one of the most interesting miracles of the human brain. It's as if the brain recognizes a break in the thought process, and it finds another path to basic problem solving.

My favorite example of this happened in early December. I smile now as I write this because in my own special way of looking at the progression of things, I see a sweetness. My husband arrived one morning to find a perplexed Walter standing in the dining room. He was flipping the light switch on and off . . . on and off . . . on and off. The switch operated the eight bulb chandelier-type lighting fixture which hung over their table. How many hours he had been standing there attempting to turn on the lights was better left unknown. On this particular morning, nothing was happening as Walter attempted his simple task. It was apparent that a fuse had blown out.

My husband began the process of switch flipping for himself. He went to the basement to check and change fuses.

This in itself was a task because usually one can holler to the person upstairs to relay back which lights were going on where. After numerous unsuccessful requests and issuing repeated directions from the basement, David made his way back upstairs deciding it was better to check for himself. David let out a long sigh as he found Walter looking for the "light to go on" in his cereal box. David just shook his head and walked away.

After deciding the fuses were okay, David began disassembling the switch unit to check connections and the next thing you know, wires were being pulled from the wall to be checked. These were fifty-year-old wires and my husband was always worried about a possible fire. David decided a trip to the hardware store was in order and returned with a new switch. Walter watched patiently as his son carefully installed it but still no luck. After what seemed to be several hours of trying to find the problem, poor David gave up. This is something he rarely does but the frustration was just taking its toll for that morning. He put all the wires back into the wall and reassembled the switch. He stood there for a moment and suddenly a ridiculous idea popped into his head. He climbed onto the table, reached up and gave a bulb a turn. "Let there be light!" . . . and the bulb went on. Around the fixture he went, giving each bulb a tiny turn until they were all lit.

It seems that the night before, we had given Dad his dinner and went home without turning off the lights. We never gave it a thought because that one lone switch had been in the same spot for all those fifty years. Apparently Dad could not find the switch, or could not remember that the switch operated the lights. Walter's perplexed mind only knew that he must turn off the lights. His brain bypassed this dilemma of the whole wall switch issue and came up with a "Plan B" so he could complete his important task.

drove home to pick up Mom's clothes which I had dropped off at the dry cleaners a couple of days before her death. She wanted to be buried in the dress she wore almost twenty years before, the dress she wore to our wedding.

# X

# Three Wishes Granted

More than a year has passed since that awful night. I can still remember how the sun was rising as I drove home, just like it was any other morning. I just needed to be alone. I reflected on Mom who had just died that night before and how she tried to show us the beautiful Angel who she saw standing by her bed. I looked as hard as I could. I wanted to see the Angel too, but I couldn't. In the end, she trusted me. She had thought for a long time before she asked me to make her three promises. Just three simple requests . . . I can do that. The first two promises seemed do-able at the time and the third, the third was easy. It just seemed to go without saying. I agreed to all three without hesitation.

Anne was a beautiful woman and always had been in my opinion. I came across many photos of her in her younger years and she was very pretty. Even now as a seventy-five-year-old woman, she was very particular about her appearance and was still quite beautiful to me. As ill as she was, she always made the journey to her hairdresser's home every other week to have her hair set. I had once heard something that I will always remember. It was said that if someone was young and beautiful, it was really only the luck of the draw, but if someone was old and beautiful . . . it was because they earned it. That was Anne. What a lovely thought. Her deep love for Walter was so evident and was something I had always admired and respected, but never fully understood until she was gone.

Anne had been very ill for the six months prior to her death. The cancer had progressed rapidly with no hope left for recovery. Our very compassionate and respected family doctor had delivered the bad news. The last several months of her life were agonizing as I watched this beautiful woman deteriorate physically more and more each day. Her once beautiful features had faded away and she now wore a face of anguish and pain. She bravely spelled out the details of her own funeral wishes.

She chose her own casket and clothes. She gave quite a bit of thought before choosing her pallbearers. This was very important to her. Those chosen few probably did not realize how much she cared for and appreciated each of them for very special and unique reasons. She wanted her stone to be made of pink granite, and described in detail how she would like it cut. She even picked out her favorite flowers for the occasion. White Calla Lilies . . . had to be White Calla Lilies, and plenty of them.

I wrote down all that she told me and I wondered if she knew, as hard as it must have been for her, what an extraordinary gift she was giving her family by making the decisions for them when it came to this. She wanted a wake, but it was important to her that she did not go out looking terrible. Promise Number One—She asked me to go to the funeral home a little early, and if she did not look as she did prior to her illness, to make sure the casket was closed. I felt I already knew the answer to this one and sadly I agreed to honor her request.

Promise Number Two—Anne had various mementos and small personal items that she wished to be delivered to special friends and family members after her death. I searched the house for each item in the weeks prior to her death. I carefully cleaned, boxed each treasure with tissue paper and wrapped each item with love. I bought her a special box of note cards. When she was having a good day, I would get out the note cards and she would write a small personal message to each of her special friends. I attached the cards to the small packages of love. As I watched the pile of packages grow in my living room each day, I knew that they were going to be delivered soon.

Promise Number Three—She looked straight into my eyes, and asked me to make sure that we took care of Dad. I gasped, and reassured her without question or hesitation that we would. I would never let anything bad happen to Dad and I promised her I would always be there for him. She knew that I loved him. She looked peaceful, and within a day or two, the hospice nurse and the priest were at the house. We as a family went to her side to tell her that it was okay to let go. I was relieved that she died at home, right where she wanted to be with her husband and children at her side.

Looking back now, I made a mental note to myself to never ask someone to honor my deathbed wishes. I decided to take care of my own final wishes as best I could in advance. All the love and good intentions can not fix certain things or prepare us for what lies ahead. Sometimes we make promises. Sometimes we fail. What is important is that we do our best. I quietly decided that I would not let anyone I loved have to carry a burden of guilt for failure if they had tried their best.

We bumbled our way through the wake and funeral on auto pilot. Going through the motions one step at a time, with no real thought of tomorrow. I remember drawing a deep breath as I walked into the funeral home. I went early as instructed. Images of how she looked that night she died etched into my brain. I remember mentally preparing my request to close the casket as promised. And then, I remember slowly approaching her casket. I stopped, I was standing there shocked . . . big giant sigh of relief . . . oh my God, how absolutely lovely she looked. The pain and anguish had vanished from her face and she truly looked years younger. Her hair was beautiful, and she was sporting that beautiful dress she wore so many years ago. She was wearing her pearls.

Now, to anyone who knows me, I have this little pet peeve about people at wakes. Without fail, someone is always gazing into the casket saying "My . . . doesn't Johnny look great!" I always cast them a disparaging look as if to say, "Great??? . . . what kind of a thing is that to say . . . for God's sake . . . he's dead." How I have changed. There I was, remarking over and over again at how absolutely beautiful she looked. She was at peace. I smiled, as I knew that Anne was probably standing there right beside me saying the exact same thing. She would have approved. Promise Number One—Mission accomplished.

The lines of well wishers came and went. I only remember pulling Walter from the casket as he wept uncontrollably. He just wanted to climb right in there with her and would not stop touching her lifeless body, stroking her hair. We again pulled ourselves together for the funeral the following day. I was angry with the three sons again. It seemed that no one thought it at all important to write a eulogy for their mother for church. Jackie said he thought David was supposed to do it as he was the oldest. David said Ray was supposed to do it as Ray was supposed to organize the church part of it. Ray said he thought that was the job of the Funeral Director. The Funeral Director? . . . . A man we had only met a couple of days ago was supposed to whip up loving words to reflect the entire life of a woman he had never met? Idiot Men . . . When someone going to put a woman in charge?

A frantic priest arrived at the funeral home, moments before we were getting ready to leave for church. He was trying to extract bits of information from the three of them about their mother's life. He desperately needed something to say about her in church. I don't really remember too much, although the priest's impromptu speech about Anne was interesting to me. "Give . . . give . . . give . . . that's what Anne's life was all about . . . give . . . give . . . give . . ." He was clearly winging it and he was sweating. Oh yes . . . he called her by the wrong name once.

I felt that pain again, shooting from my neck down my back and down my right leg. Maybe no one else noticed his slight error. I was sitting in the front pew of the church clinging to Walter's arm. Words . . . music . . . more words . . . Amen. I just couldn't seem to concentrate. What I do remember came at the very end. As people were leaving, one by one I asked Anne's special friends to follow me to the car.

One by one I handed them their very special gifts and cards from Anne. Their sad faces, at first shocked and puzzled at seeing her handwriting, beamed a wonderful glow as they read their special message from Anne. They all cried, they all smiled, they all laughed. Their heads shook in disbelief and glowed with happiness because Anne had taken time to remember them in such a special way. As they walked away clutching their personal treasure, in some very small way . . . maybe it was a big way . . . I don't know, I watched them begin to heal. I will never be able to describe what a true privilege and very rare gift it was for me to be chosen to carry out Promise Number Two. Mission accomplished.

The sympathy cards, fruit baskets, flowers, casseroles and support came with a fury those first few days. I would sit with Walter every night and read each card, each message several times out loud. All of those words of kindness really meant a lot to him. It seemed that all of this ended abruptly after only a week. I'm not sure what I expected. I guess I was hoping the cards would still keep coming in great mounds until we were all just a little better. You know . . . like for the next year or two until we could start feeling like we could somehow move on again. It was a very lonely time. I thought to myself to always remember what it felt like during that time. I made a promise that if someone I knew had died, to make sure that I did something nice for the family in the weeks and even the months that followed. It was important to let them know that they were not forgotten, long after the cards and flowers had stopped arriving.

We again were drawing on Joan's love and support during those tough times and for the even tougher times ahead. She had such love for her big brother, Walter. She supported David and loved him like he was her son. She loved me too. She also supported us as the tough decisions were being made. She eased the guilt, and there was plenty of guilt brewing up inside ourselves these days. Many people had showered us with praise for the great job we did caring for both Mom and Dad, but I guess we saw only our failings. I was thinking that if these well wishers could have only seen us in action, falling apart and losing control so many, many times. It was praise we did not deserve.

Now a year later, one chilly winter afternoon, a neighbor up the street called David at work and told him that he had noticed Walter wandering around the Shopping Village that day. He said he saw him again a little while later up the road from his house. When talking to him, Walter wasn't sure where he was going and this friend drove him back to his home. A relative called that same day to say that Walter had just crossed the four lane highway near his house and cars were beeping and swerving to avoid hitting him.

We arrived at Dad's house in a panic, to find a very quiet Walter sitting in his big chair with his cat. We asked Dad what he had been doing that day, and he told us he had pretty much been sitting there, just petting Jake. He told us he was watching a show on TV about a man with Alzheimer's Disease. He told us that if he were that man, he would just pick the coldest day of the year and go for a walk. He would go for a long walk . . . and he would just keep on walking. My thoughts immediately flashed back to that poor woman I had been told about who wall papered her father's doors. I could picture her crying in lonely desperation as she fumbled through her tool box as she relocated all of the doorknobs.

Our faces went white. My Promise . . . Promise Number Three, to take care of Dad. I could hear Anne's voice shrieking at me inside my head to take care of Dad. Where were those "friends" now . . . the ones who had repeatedly told us that Dad was "perfectly fine," "just like the old days," "remembered every detail," "maybe we were just over reacting." My thoughts were interrupted by David. "Janet . . . " he said sadly, "get me the phone." Our world was about to change again. This time in a big way. I was not going to need my tool box.

# XI
## Shady Pines

There were a number of facilities in the area, all shapes, all sizes, all outwardly cheerful and all inwardly grim. David and his brothers had visited a number of facilities in the area earlier that fall, and returned home with sad stories of the residents and their daily routine. We had decided on a newly built facility which was dedicated to the care of specifically Alzheimer's residents. The facility was quite nice and the staff was wonderful from what I could observe. It was clean and the calendar of planned daily activities for the residents was very impressive. The beautiful and very cheerful shell of the facility masked the true tragedy and reality of the lives of the residents inside. In comparison with the others, Dad seemed much more aware than most of the residents and his condition was considered "mild." We could look around and easily see what was in store for us by the interaction with residents more advanced.

Each room was private and each had their own bathroom. The room was simply but cheerfully decorated. A long high shelf ran along the side wall. I noticed that other residents had framed photographs and other assorted memorabilia neatly lined up on their shelves. Outside each door hung a shadow box, where family members assembled mementoes and photos of the resident's life. Their life's story all summed up in a tidy framed box. In the months to come,

I would spend many hours getting to know the various residents on whatever level I could. I enjoyed looking at every detail of each of their shadow boxes and appreciated them for the lives they represented before this disease took away their treasured memories. Could it be that only the shadows of their previous existence remained? . . . Those far away memories were left only as shadows now, and they faded for each of those poor souls a little more each day.

A facility social worker had visited Dad's home a month earlier. It was an interview of sorts, assessing his condition I guess to see if he was eligible to be put on the list. The process seemed strange to me and I'm sure, as I have done so many times before, I have misinterpreted the whole thing. First of all, one needs money, and plenty of it. Rule number one . . . they are private companies of sorts, not considered nursing homes, and not mandated to accept Title 19. You are a resident in good standing as long as you still have cash and as long as your condition does not require extensive special care. Apparently, as one's condition advances, they are required to be moved to a nursing home. Hmmmm . . . so far I'm not on board with this. I am not getting that warm fuzzy feeling they want you to get when they show their TV commercials of your aging parent skipping through the daisies at their facility.

I also felt that Dad needed to be advanced enough to fit into the surroundings, yet not advanced to the point of agitation where he would be considered a threat to others, or a constant irritation to the staff. I paced back and forth and wrung my hands, hoping Dad would "pass" the tests. I let out a huge sigh of relief as the facility worker announced that he would indeed be eligible . . . oh yes . . . and that she thought that Walter was a very nice man. I momentarily felt that rush of pride, you know, like hearing the news that your kid passed the test and was accepted into college. Wait a minute, this is not that, back to reality. It was time to step back and become the adult . . . I hate that. We had become too close to the situation, too caught up in emotion. We were overcome with the guilty feelings that come with sneaking around the back of your loved one, planning that dastardly scheme where you whisk them off to the home. Do you tell him or do you not? When do you do it? How do you do it?

The books are full of suggestions. The books are filled with knowledge. The library shelf is growing with books. They say help is abundant, information resources growing in leaps and bounds. The web is flooded with new information as I already knew. It is now after midnight. I wonder where these esteemed writers are now. I'm thinking they are tucked safely away in there little beds sleeping peacefully. I have a headache and I no longer sleep. I have got to get up early for work tomorrow, I mean today. How do we possibly break the news to Dad? I think we are going to wing it this time. I am tired of reading the books. I rummaged through the drawer hoping I have not used the last of the Tylenol.

I had really hoped that all three of Walter's sons could have been there on moving day. To me, it would have been a symbolic gesture of unity, supporting Dad with one strong father-son bond of unanimous support, everyone in agreement for the sake, safety and care of Walter. There was something about brothers helping brothers too. Doing it together may have lessened the guilt, or maybe just redistributed the guilt three ways, I guess. That didn't happen in the way I would have liked, but it couldn't be helped, I guess. David and his brother Ray took Dad for a ride to his new home. We opted not to tell him in advance as we were all concerned after his comment about going for a walk and never coming back.

53

We did not exactly trick him, I mean we didn't coax him into the car with promises of an ice cream cone. He was simply told that we wanted him to try out this new apartment, where there would be people there who would help him. I'm not sure that this was the right thing to do, but you can only make the best decisions you can at the moment you need to make them. Dad had no idea he was leaving his home for good that morning but he went quietly and accepted their decision. Dad issued a brief instruction to Jake to guard the place. David and Ray watched quietly as he bent down to lovingly pat his cat's head, Walter struggled with the zipper on his coat and then they left. That was it.

Walter was greeted by a warm waiting staff on the other end. I stayed away that morning. I went to work like it was any other day, guarding my private self and doing my job. I was haunted by incredible guilt that I had somehow betrayed this man whom I loved. I have always been the emotional type. I take things to heart, maybe a little too much, but that's who I am. I knew I would cry if I were there and more than anything, I could not bear to have him look at me with hurt in his eyes.

The staff had instructed us on the positive behavior we needed to convey during the initial period especially, and I was not strong enough to keep my emotions upbeat and perky as they requested. David, Raymond and Raymond's son moved Dad in. They brought Dad's favorite chair, his bed and dresser, his favorite selection of photos, clothes and a clock. They left him with the coordinator who took him under her wing, introducing him to all the residents.

After work that day, I asked David to take me back there so I could see how he was doing for myself. The staff suggested that we do not visit for the first week or so, I guess so that Walter could become acclimated with the people and his new environment. What did they mean . . . not a good idea to visit? Of course I had other ideas and by now my mind was filled with all kinds of visions of horrible goings-on at that place. I wanted to see what was really going on once the family had dropped off their loved one. David assured me that all would be okay, but after persistent requests, eventually he agreed to take me.

Now, all I can say in my own defense is that long periods of stress can make relatively sane individuals do strange things. It was nightfall when we arrived and I found myself in the bushes of the place peering in through the window of Dad's room. I just had to see for myself how he was being treated when the staff thought no one was watching. I wondered if they had security cameras out here? By now I was in a state of fear and fully prepared to open my can of whoop-ass if anyone was in any way harming him. Damn . . . .he's not in his room.

Well, there is always Plan B . . . I guess I can try being an adult again and actually go inside. Where did I put the code to gain access to this place? The contents of my purse fell in the bushes. Now I'm groping in the dark in the bushes to retrieve my stuff, expecting at any moment to hear the sounds of alarms and experience the blinding beam of security floodlights. My brain is frantically organizing my explanation speech. Hmmmm . . . No alarms . . . no blinding lights . . . perhaps I have escaped humiliation undetected.

I punched in the code at the door of this lock-down facility and I quietly crept down the corridor. I could hear Dad's voice coming from the community gathering room in his wing . . . . Wait a minute . . . he is laughing!! . . . and talking!! I stood out of sight around the corner and just listened. He was busy charming the staff in that very special way he had. I carefully peeked around the corner. One nurse had already nicknamed him "Mr. B" and she had her arm around his shoulders, as she was introducing him to other residents.

I could see his big smile as he was introducing himself. He never saw me, and I quietly left. David and I didn't talk at all on the long drive home, but I heard myself utter "Thank You, God" many times. I wasn't quite sure if God was listening or if he was in approval of our actions that day. All of the home-alone safety issues plagued me for many months before, and I agreed with the decisions made to bring him here. I am just hoping we haven't overlooked another kinder alternative, whatever that might be.

The book said that relief may or may not be the expected reaction after a relative has been moved. So far I agree. We may feel enormous relief that others are involved in the care and supervision of our loved one, or we may not feel relief at all because it is often difficult to share the care with other caregivers. No . . . sharing is good and I'm okay with that. Or we may feel relief quickly followed by guilt. Yah . . . that's it . . . relief quickly followed by guilt. I thought about Mom and I waited for that giant lightning bolt to come from the sky and hit me. Nothing happened. I thought again about "Maggie," She never would have dumped her loved one at a facility or nursing home and I am not too proud of myself right now. I have a lot more thinking to do about the whole thing, but for right now, I will go home and assemble seventy-six years of wonderful memories into one small shadow box.

# XII

## Stuck in a Loop

The staff all seemed to love Dad. Who wouldn't after all, he was charming and polite and they described him as a leader after only a few days. Every time we arrived, it seemed he had a small parade of other residents lined up and following him up and down the halls. One staff member said she just loved him and he reminded her of her own Dad. Those few words were a great comfort and he seemed to be adjusting well. Things changed after a few weeks. We would arrive to find Dad, all packed, just sitting there with his hat and coat on. He was sad. He wanted to go home.

The book said that this was "normal." Now there was good news. It was "normal" for our loved one to feel sad and lost with a sense of not belonging. He was not comfortable with his surroundings, with community activities or any social situations in his new home. The book said that often families feel so much guilt and are so anxious for their relative to be happy in his new home that they try and talk him out of feelings of anger, sadness or denial. This is bad apparently, and we should discontinue this type of behavior immediately.

It said we must allow Dad to experience his feelings and say things like "I can see you are feeling sad" and then we are supposed to hold his hand. It is "normal" and necessary for him to experience all of these feelings and emotions.

Again I am wondering just who writes this stuff anyway? Is their father crying for the first time ever right in front of them, begging for help, and begging them to just take him home?

The book said that it is quite common for our loved one to feel relieved when they are moved. Often they are lost and lonely with no sense of purpose and have felt that they were a burden to their family or care giver, or they had begun to feel unsafe or bored in their old environment. For some people, there was great security in having people around and a routine to follow. The book said that sometimes our relatives can surprise us with a totally different reaction than we expect. The book says that some residents are excited by their new environment. Those who have been used to living alone may be overwhelmed by the number of people and things to do, but also excited by them. Bull . . . I am looking around and am not seeing this excitement they speak of in any face here.

David would unpack Dad's things and explain again to Walter that he would have to stay there for a while, as these people were going to help him. Walter was having increased trouble expressing himself, but would convey stories of strange goings-on in the place. All night long it seems, people were taking his belongings, furniture and clothes, and were loading them in trucks out back to make off with them. David would show Dad that all of his belongings were in order and Dad would state that they must be bringing his things back by morning, so that outsiders wouldn't catch on.

Dad wanted his car. He said he was leaving and began developing escape plans. I noticed that I was becoming increasingly irritated with David. He would at times become stern with Dad and as Dad spoke, slowly and with broken thought patterns as he tried to explain something, David would jump in and finish all of his sentences. Dad was troubled and very frustrated. He would stutter and cry. "The loop . . . it's the loop" he would start to say, but couldn't go any further.

David would jump in "you must mean the loop on your trousers. Dad, your pants are fine, don't worry about it." Walter would agree with David every time, as David was telling him what he meant or how he felt. I could see by the look on Walter's face that he really had much more to say. We began to argue on the way home. I could feel Walter's frustration and confusion and I accused David of not taking the time to listen.

I felt as though Walter, who was really struggling with communicating, would sometimes speak with puzzling references. Much of it did not make sense the first time around. Maybe if we did a better job at just being quiet, we could understand the method to his madness. I remembered his unique problem solving abilities which he displayed at home. If he could not get the job done in the traditional manner, he would find a roundabout way to complete his task. There was something we were missing here. It was something big and important.

My mind shifted to thoughts of Grandpa, Walter's father. He was another wonderful man and clearly, the apple hadn't fallen far from the tree. It had to be at least eighteen years earlier. Grandpa was dying of cancer and was spending his last few precious days in the hospital. The end was grueling, and he was on pain medication. Family had visited and he would ramble on and on about how there were loud parties going on all night long and the train was rumbling past his door at all hours of the night keeping him awake. We would just bob our heads in agreement and give each other quiet looks on the side. That medication was really working his reality.

One night near the end, David and I decided to visit him. We ended up staying and eventually dozed off in chairs. Sometime in the wee hours, I was awoken abruptly by the sound of laughter. Grandpa's room was right near the nurse's station, and there was some kind of a big hoop-la going on. *What the hell,* I thought, *is there a party going on down there?* I listened to my own words. The next thing I heard was the loud rumble of some kind of a large laundry cart rattling its way down the corridor. Damned if it didn't sound just like a train. Grandpa taught me one last valuable lesson that night before he left us.

I decided to visit Walter one night after work on my own. I arrived to find sad Dad sitting in his room, with hat and coat on, things all packed. He was confused and upset, and putting together the pieces of conversation became more difficult when he was upset. I simply asked him what was wrong, and then I sat in silence. He began talking about "the loop." He was agitated and could not describe what the loop meant. My initial reaction was to jump right in there and help him out, tell him what I thought it meant. I could tell him anything and he would agree, then we could talk about the weather. It seemed the kind thing to do as it is almost like torture watching a loved one struggle so much trying to get the message across.

This loop thing was really important to him. Instead, I sat there with my mouth closed and my eyes fixed on his upset face. He looked at me with that handsome face for a long time as we sat in silence. "Dad," I said softly, "tell me about the loop." He started and stopped, started and stopped. I sat quietly and just listened. When he got stuck, he would stop and start over again. Eventually, I believed he understood that I was listening, and that I was not leaving until he had said what he had been so desperately trying to communicate.

He slowly began by explaining that the people who were taking care of him were very nice. Typical Dad, always a kind word, and always appreciative. He looked at me, almost embarrassed or ashamed. "I'm in trouble," he said softly. "I'm in real trouble and for the first time in my life I just don't know what to do." He started to cry. He explained how he had always taken care of himself, his family and how he had always tried to do the right thing. Somehow he had landed himself in this place, but he couldn't remember signing up for it.

He told me that he was always responsible for his actions, but this time he really made a big mistake. He said he has been asking everyone why he was here and what was he going to do while he was here, but no one would answer. He wanted to know the plan and no one would answer him. He wanted to know what his job was here and no one would answer him. My heart broke.

He said he had spent many hours of each day, trying to replay the series of events that happened to him over the past several weeks. As he described his torment, I could almost hear an old scratched record playing in my head as he spoke. It was like that old scratched and broken record was replaying the same short bar of words and music over and over again, then it would skip back to the same starting spot. Each time you hope the song will continue, but it doesn't. It skips back to that same spot and starts over.

He was desperately trying to understand how his actions had landed him in this place. He was desperately trying to understand how his actions could have gotten him into so much trouble. He told me that he goes to sleep each night and replays it over and over again. He said it's like he's stuck in a loop that he can't get out of. He said that only weeks ago his life was fine, and he needed to go back home. He needed to go back to his job and take care of his cat and

61

his garden. The pain was so clearly evident as he had been torturing himself over and over again.

He was struggling over and over again, trying to recollect how his decisions could have landed him in so much trouble. He was blaming himself for the decisions we had made to protect and care for him. I listened carefully and patiently as he struggled even more to find the words to explain his anguish of being stuck in this never ending loop. Suddenly, I understood perfectly what he was saying and feeling. I hugged him hard and told him just that. He cried and thanked me. A look of genuine relief swept across his face.

I told him that I was going to call David to come over so we could all talk about what he was feeling. I felt we had not given him enough credit or explanation on the plan here, and I knew he was blaming himself and was suffering. I was busy blaming ourselves for failing to carry out this very important move with more care. We were participants in events which were hurting Walter. I told him that no matter what, I would always be there for him and that I loved him. We all loved him, and we would help him. This amazing man found his own way to communicate and get the job done once again.

I spent that night tossing and turning in my bed, staring up at the ceiling fan and thinking. God, we are so not qualified. Our handling of things has now caused this poor man to blame himself. Hurting him was not part of Promise Number Three. I replayed his explanation of "the loop" over and over again, trying to remember each and every word as he explained it. That very moment in time, that moment when I understood his anguish of the loop, is a moment I will not forget. In an instant it struck home very hard for me.

Several years earlier, a young person and someone I loved very much had gone away to college. He was chock full of promise with his whole wonderful life ahead of him. He was one great individual. Then he became involved with drugs, which led to a series of terrible events. Each event worse than the previous and in an instant, changed and hurt the lives of many people. My life was not just changed . . . my life was destroyed. A close friend of his arrived at our home one day. He was worried and I could tell he was upset. He had tried to confide the extent of the problem to me a year earlier. It must have been very difficult for him. Those two were more like brothers and had been friends since they were both five years old.

I didn't listen. I was in denial. I was the adult and if something like that was going on, I surely would have been the first one to recognize the problem. The problems quickly began to accelerate out of control. It wasn't until everything was in chaos that I tried to fling myself into the middle of it to stop the madness. I tried to get help in many different ways. I spent days at the hospital by his bedside, begging doctors and God for help. Interventions did not work. I quickly retreated into my own very small world.

I was frantic and consumed with fear. I was embarrassed too, and I found myself uncomfortable and walking around with my head down for fear of running into someone who knew even more of the details than I did. I guess as I felt that I would be judged by the havoc this individual was wreaking around town. I stopped answering the phone. I wouldn't even go to the grocery store anymore. I wouldn't go to the mailbox either as I would find upsetting correspondence informing me of more problems.

I spent my waking hours trying to function at work, always in a secret panic, terrified that the phone would ring, always with more terrible news. I would go to sleep, and have the same bad recurring dream. It was quite vivid and always ended in death. I would replay all the events over and over again in my dream, trying desperately to get back to the time when things were good. Rewriting the events in my head to somehow change the ending. I had read somewhere that dreams were a great fount of knowledge, just waiting to be tapped. I couldn't find the knowledge that I needed to understand what had happened. I felt incredible guilt. I should have done this . . . I should have done that . . . I was in this terrible loop that just kept replaying like a bad movie that wouldn't end. No matter what I did, I couldn't change the ending. I reached out to someone very close to me for help, but that person did not or could not hear me.

I only wanted to hear those wonderful words . . . . "I understand." It was a very lonely world. It was a loop which lasted almost seven years. As hope faded, I finally decided that there had to be a reason. Please God, let there be a reason. I must have been meant to experience my own loop so that I might be able to help someone else though it. The circumstances were very different but the feelings were the same. I would be able to understand the sorrow, desperation and fear by experiencing it firsthand. I was sure I would be empathetic toward others because of it. Walter, I will not let you down and you are not alone. I'm going to find a way to help you break the loop.

# XIII
# Shhhhhhh . . . I'm Trying to Listen

It's amazing to me that I have lived so many years and I
never learned to listen. I decided that the problem with the
world today is that too many people really enjoy the sound
of their own voice. They are so impressed with their gift that
they feel it is to our benefit if they share their vast knowledge
of the world regularly. Think about it for a moment. How
many people do you know at work or personally, where you
could honestly say that the lives of everyone around them
would be much better served if that person gave a little more
thought to listening instead of blessing us all with their views
on every topic. Usually I find that what they lack in knowledge, they will simply make up for in volume. I'm smiling
as my list pops into my head. I'm making another mental
note to myself . . . practice active listening, I just might learn
something, and I might be a little less annoying to those
around me.

This new approach is working so well when communicating with Walter. Although this basic concept of listening
may be so obvious to others, it somehow escaped our little
family unit. Walter seems much less frustrated to me. He
continues to start expressing his thoughts and fades off. Now
I don't let him off the hook. I continue to fix my gaze on
his face until he is satisfied that he is all done. Even if the
thought is not clear to me. If he is all done and satisfied

then so am I. Oh yes . . . I hold his hand while he talks as instructed by the book. The book was right.

One thing is still bothering him though. He is very worried about money. He is always checking his wallet and asks how he is going to pay for this place. He is worried sick that someone is going to hand him a bill and he won't know what to do. We keep reassuring him that everything was okay, and he didn't have to worry at all about paying any bills.

David had been handling his finances for several years now, and Dad never worried about any money matters, so I wasn't quite sure where this was coming from. Some of the other more vocal residents would angrily express their feelings about the cost of the place, and maybe he overheard their discussions and worries. I don't know. We told him he was in good shape and not to worry about a thing. This discussion was repeated almost daily for about two weeks. Then one day, out of the blue, Dad cheerfully announced to us that his apartment, his food and even his haircuts were free! He was very excited about this. We weren't quite sure what had happened, we just smiled and nodded anyway. Dad never questioned the money issue again.

I was proud of Dad's shadow box. I had gone through at least a thousand family photographs, looking for those special few which would show the world just how wonderful this man was. The largest photograph was a beautiful old sepia wedding portrait. He and Anne were both just twenty-one when they married and that photo was a classic. I placed that in the center of the box, as Anne would have wanted it that way.

I picked out my personal favorite photo of Walter as a child. It was his First Holy Communion, and he was dressed in his tidy knickers and pressed shirt. He also wore a tie. His hair was neatly combed. For the photo, his mother had posed him reverently with his hands pressed together in a praying position, but the twinkle in his eye was that of a boy who wanted to fling his tie in the bushes and run off to play baseball with his friends.

I also found several great pictures of Walter with his brother and sister as children, standing in front of the old family car. I found nice pictures of his parents too. The photos progressed with pictures of him as a young Navy man, and the Naval Cruiser on which he served. Later, in his twenties, as he worked for his Dad at a Studebaker dealership. Later, in his thirties, as the owner of his own garage and car dealership, and later than that, when he was in his forties, where he worked with explosives for a Drilling and Blasting company and where he was known throughout the state as the "Master Blaster."

The shadow box contained photos of his three sons, and his grandchildren, holidays, family parties and vacations to Maine. It displayed photos of his very close friends who had always been by his side since they all were young. There were pictures of him working, fishing and selling his raspberries. There were pictures of his Studebaker sign and pictures of his blasting signs. There was a picture of the racing stock car which was sponsored by his garage business. There were pictures of his garden. I carefully assembled the pictures and decided I needed to add a few of his personal items for him to look at in the years to come.

I got out my hot melt glue gun and attached his favorite fishing lures and flies, his fishing license, his favorite spark plug tie tack, his business cards from his garage business and also from the drilling and blasting company he worked for. I glued in his lucky Indian arrowhead from Maine and last but not least, I glued in a small gold colored trophy which I had attached to his Father's Day gift one year which read "World's Greatest Dad." All of these items were assembled with love and I knew that it was a fitting tribute, and a clear representation of a hard-working man with a wide variety of interests. It also represented a man who was always surrounded by a loving family. His shadow box was filled with as many of his life's details as I could jam in there. I carefully cleaned the glass and proudly hung it on the wall outside his room.

My mind began searching for more answers as I looked at his life from behind the glass. Was there something in these pictures which held the answer? Maybe there was a link. During his many years spent working at the garage, I'm sure he was exposed to toxins and chemicals. It was common practice to wash various auto parts, and one's own hands in gasoline . . . leaded gasoline. I examined his blasting photos. He spent many years exposed to various blasting agents. Many of the other resident shadow boxes contained old military photos, just like Dad's. In his youth, Dad worked on farms and could have been exposed to now-banned pesticides. I wondered if all of these shadow boxes up and down the halls held a secret in common.

A month has passed and Dad seems to be settled in. He says he doesn't eat very much but to me it looks as if he has gained twenty pounds. He looks great and has even started singing "Zippity-do-dah" again. For a while there, he was always asking for explicit directions to get him to the parking lot. He would look out of his window and ask which way he should turn once he got to the end of the driveway. He was no longer packing up his things and refers to his new place as his home. We have not yet taken him out for an outing as we want to make sure it will not be an upsetting ordeal getting him back.

Maybe we will give him a couple more weeks and then we'll take him out for lunch or ice cream and see what happens. He had not mentioned his beloved "Jake" once since that night of explaining the loop. We even got special permission from the supervisors here to have Jake come for a visit if Dad asked. I had been so worried about tearing him away from his cat, yet for nearly a month, not a word . . . nothing. And don't think I am not listening for those little subliminal clues because I am and I'll be on them like lightning this time.

Then one day out of the blue, Dad said he had the strangest dream. He dreamed his cat was on his bed and he woke up worried. He looked for Jake and Jake was gone. He wanted to know where his cat was and if he was okay. We assured Dad that Jake was fine and well taken care of. We even showed Dad the picture of his cat we had in his night stand. Walter seemed a little baffled as he studied the photo. He put the picture back in the drawer and never mentioned him again. He never asked about his house or his garden. He was beginning to ask about Anne. Where was she, was she at this house, things like that. By now it's been about a year and a half since she died but I believe he is starting to search the place for her.

I had read somewhere that a woman had to keep telling her aging parent over and over again that the spouse had passed away, which caused the remaining parent to grieve over and over again. Each time shocked at the news of the death of their loved one. That is one terrible loop to relive. I keep asking God why these poor souls can't just be stuck in the loop of their greatest and happiest day of their life. That little voice came back to me gently saying "keep listening girlfriend . . . you have so much more to learn about life." It appears I may have to live to be a hundred before I get a clue.

# XIV

# See You Later

Dad was safe, but the stress on our end did not go away, it simply shifted in a whole different direction. David was trying to rebuild his own shrinking business, and the focus was now shifting from role of care giver to elderly parents to more of life's issues. David was a good man and a great son. I did not want to push him but we really needed to press on with the sale of Dad's house. No one really wanted to sell it. It meant that this life's change was now permanent. David would continue to postpone moving forward, always saying "There is no hurry, we can do this later." David was also handling the probate stuff and the settling of Mom's estate. Her records were a mess. He was in charge of contacting the insurance companies, inventory of her assets, requesting bank statements and processing the transfer and sale of stock. Papers were everywhere.

Dealing with the sale of the house, removal of old oil tanks, the disposition of any items to family or for sale to support Dad were now at the top of the list. The big black Buick needed to be sold. Dealing with environmental lawyers and the sale of commercial properties owned by Walter as an LLC, keeping books on rental property, appointments with accountants and realtors were next on the list. These things were followed by meetings with special Elder Care Attorneys, calling estate auctioneers, and hiring dumpsters.

The list went on and on. His Dad's rental property always had problems which needed immediate attention. David was always the one to drop what he was doing and fix whatever was wrong.

The worst part was the cleaning of this little house which sheltered every piece of paper and memento accumulated for over fifty years. Every closet, cupboard, nook and cranny jammed to the ceiling. The upstairs had two bedrooms, each now packed, every inch with junk, even broken junk. It was a huge undertaking. We had many discussions with Mom and Dad, asking them to start getting rid of some of the stuff accumulated over the years and they indignantly refused. This was their stuff, and no one was going to tell them what to do. It now became our problem. Bag upon bag upon bag was filled, most of which found its way to the dumpster or to the auctioneer. The meager rest, which was later reduced to several boxes of tag sale items, were all that was left. Amazing, fifty plus years of accumulating these treasures. Now they sit unceremoniously in a cardboard box in the garage.

I was trying my best to support David, while at the same time working, trying not to panic as I was again worried if my paycheck could support our mortgage payment. I have to say that this was beginning to grind on me as the months were apparently turning into years. We would argue as I felt that his siblings needed to help out more. He told me that he felt that it was his ''job in life'' to take care of his parents, and that his brothers had their own lives to lead, families to raise, and jobs to go to. Each had their own worries and responsibilities to attend to. His brother Ray, and his family lived out of town and helped out as best as they could, and the youngest brother Jackie and his family lived in Florida. What were they supposed to do? I didn't know the answer to that question, but to be honest, I wanted to see a little more long-distance suffering perhaps.

Here's the part where I am going to hell . . . I was not buying this any longer. Everyone needed to pitch in. Was anyone else concerned that all of this has now caused us financial hardship because David was not working? David was still self-employed and had his own business to run, but the calls began to dwindle again because he was never there. Our bank account was shrinking more and more each month, as the mortgage still needed to be paid. Why was I not informed prior to my wedding day about his "job in life"? He needed to ask his brothers for help. I was tired and had reached my frozen limit. I was becoming ugly, a witch to be sure . . . although those I held most dear were spelling it with a "b." I did not live in Kansas, but I was scanning the sky, searching for that whirling house which I was sure would be plummeting down on me at any given moment. Just like in the movie, all that would be left of that malevolent creature was the remains of two legs, unceremoniously sticking out from under that relocated house. Shoes intact, broomstick broken.

I was wondering why they seemed, at times, lax in returning our phone calls as we were struggling. Maybe we needed help or maybe we just needed to talk. There was something missing here that I just couldn't understand or respect. David was taking on more than his fair share and I was not liking it. There was a time in my life not so very long ago when I really needed David, and he wasn't there for me. It was a very rough time, and he wasn't there. I never forgot that. I loved David and I loved David's parents, but for twenty years now I have always been aware that I have had to take a backseat to them on David's priority list.

There wasn't any what one might call sibling rivalry going on I don't think. It was all very polite and civilized for the most part. All three boys were very nice people. According to the book I was reading, some families can just be torn apart at times like these. Siblings can often have very different opinions as everyone sorts out their own priorities. My feelings of a cooperative solution were abruptly altered in one fleeting moment. It was just one little outburst which happened about a week before Mom died. It was nothing, yet it seemed huge to me. Everyone was really feeling the stress of watching Mom deteriorate as the end was near. Jackie and his family came up from Florida to help. Raymond spent several nights helping out too.

We had engaged a live-in hospice worker through the local Visiting Nurse Association. She was a very kind and diligent young woman in her mid-twenties. She came from Armenia and we had a little trouble communicating at times, but we enjoyed hearing about her home and her family. She was dedicated to her job and she gave us a lot of help and peace of mind. She would laugh as we would correct her English, and she would teach us little phrases in Armenian. I was glad that we found her. We cleaned out an upstairs room and helped her move in. She was very attentive to Mom who now summoned her continuously though the night. She loved Dad and she kept a watchful eye on him always. He was comfortable having her in the house. She was very organized and kept the little house very tidy. She was a good cook as well.

Shortly after her arrival, she came down with the flu. This was unfortunate as now she was confined to her room so as not to spread any germs. She did not have family in the area, or a place in this country which she could call home. We needed to nurse her back to health as soon as possible for our own sake. We had to pick up the ball again and I was busy bringing her soup and juice while I prayed for a speedy recovery so she could resume her caregiving. Mom was demanding. I didn't blame her of course. I'm sure I would have been someone's worse nightmare if I had been in her shoes. Our care giver got well after two long and grueling weeks and we all breathed a huge sigh of relief. Even with a live-in hospice worker, every minute seemed emotionally charged.

I was in the living room with Mom and Dad as the sons were trying to organize papers and other legal-related things in the next room. At one point, I heard an agitated voice bark at David, telling him that he was making "too big of a damned deal out of everything." My face burned. They had no clue as to how much of David's life was spent in this house helping his parents. Through good times and through bad, he was there every day, several times a day if they needed him, and they usually did. How could someone minimize everything he had done to help them by saying something so condescending? Mom and Dad had heard it too and asked me who was yelling and what was wrong. I told them it was nothing.

The words "too big of a damned deal" were etched in my brain. What we were dealing with was huge. It was really too bad that I was a lady. I could have marched in there and let loose a flood of language which I learned in the Navy that would have curled their hair. David told me to just forget it. The solution with this family was to sweep things under the carpet. I could not.

Okay . . . let's not judge everyone else as everyone is different. Everyone handles their problems in life their own way. Some people show it . . . some people don't. It didn't mean that those people didn't care, it was just their way. Well, I didn't like their way. I just wanted to know why, when we were having trouble and needed support, at times we would not even have our phone calls returned. The books say that even with a large family, the responsibility of primary care giver usually gravitates itself to one person. Swell. I already figured that one out for myself.

There were other family members outside of the immediate circle who often asked if they could help. I wasn't really sure what we could ask of them. I wasn't sure that we had a right to ask anything of them. We were all part of a very large extended family and it was not so many years ago that David's brother had a very serious health problem which required finding a bone marrow donor to save his life. I saw firsthand the unbelievable outpouring of support from not only family members and friends, but also from total strangers as well. Countless hours of people's time and money was spent doing everything and anything they could to help us. I never saw such an outpouring of support in my life.

It could only be compared to the movie *It's A Wonderful Life*. When the chips were down, it was the entire town's people who all came together for George Bailey. It demonstrated that his life had touched so many people in ways he wasn't even aware. George Bailey discovered that his life had so much meaning. He had a lovely tapestry of family, friends, neighbors and strangers. In the end, he even helped an Angel get his wings. Things like that didn't just happen in the movies, I saw it happen firsthand. I still relive the events of that horrible time, but always appreciated it as a true miracle from God that a donor was found in time. More than that, I really appreciated being part of a very large family that all rallied around when someone was in trouble. It was such a beautiful and heartwarming thing to witness. It was a real life tribute to mankind.

Our family was in trouble again, but this time it was different. It's hard to explain. I knew how much work, both physically and emotionally, was involved just getting through each day at that point. I guess I felt that asking for help was not right, until all of the immediate family was pitching in one hundred percent. Maybe I was embarrassed that we were behaving badly. The brothers were not pitching in again.

This time it was said by one of them that "They had their own life to lead." How very nice for them. As I listened, I was strangely amused as it seemed that they were convinced that they were greatly overwhelmed with doing their fair share. Why was I not seeing that?

I am thinking, no . . . I am hoping that as the years pass and the emotions settle themselves down, I will be able to look back at this with an enlightened perspective. I hope to have a greater understanding of the whole situation and am able to see things through the eyes of others. I don't like walking around like this. I am a twisted knot of emotions. I love David's brothers and they are good people. They loved their mother and they love their father.

I think that my true feelings be told, it has more to do with my own feelings of desperation, and feelings of being hurt. I feel as if no one cares enough to see that I am hurt. Of course I am not willing to reach out to anyone either. In polite society, we must not disclose the family dirty laundry, so these kinds of feelings must be kept private. This type of thinking only serves to make me a hurt, frustrated and very lonely big dummy.

One cold Sunday afternoon when Mom was still with us, we were all arguing again about responsibilities and priorities, tempers began to flare. Now we had conflict with Mom about having a hospital bed delivered to the house. We really needed that bed put in the living room of their small house to help us to take better care of her. Why was she arguing? I listened to the heated conversation and I shook my head. Every moment seemed emotionally charged. Each member of the family seemed to have their own personal agenda. We needed help. Yes, I think I . . . we were embarrassed to ask anyone for anything. We were too busy acting badly.

I needed a momentary distraction from the dysfunctional mayhem and I glanced out of the living room window. It was then that I saw Mom and Dad's nephew blowing and raking the leaves in their front yard. We didn't ask him for help, he was just out there doing it on his own. I stopped dead in my tracks as I watched. I'm not sure if I cried as I watched him doing this little act of kindness all on his own. To me, this was huge. It meant so much to me to witness such a selfless act, while we were within these walls arguing about whose responsibilities were whose. Perhaps I was judging others too harshly. Perhaps I was not being sensitive to the siblings' needs. Perhaps I was not being sensitive to their lives. I didn't really care. Were they doing the same for us?

All of that was a long time ago. Why was I feeling all of these things now? I became more and more upset and I wasn't exactly sure why. David certainly had his hands full and I was feeling selfish. It seemed like a bad time for me to start having my own problems, yet I knew something bad, something really bad was brewing. I was holding a lot of hurt, anger and confusion deep inside. I tried to talk to David. He just offhandedly told me to talk to a priest, or maybe join a support group. I didn't want to talk to a priest. Despite all the wonderful testimonials I had read from people who had joined various groups, I would not go. I was losing ground. This did not happen overnight. This had been going on for some time.

To make matters worse, the company I had worked for, over the past several years, was going through a merger. It seemed as though I was working night and day to assure myself of job security. I loved my job and my life was my job, so I thought. As the company was being dismantled, I was given a new position with my salary, retirement and benefits all intact. I even got a spiffy new title and brand new business cards which read "Financial Accounting Specialist." That should make up for the extra four hours a day I spent grinding my teeth commuting in rush hour traffic.

The bad news was I would have to relocate. David was not about to sell the house and move. This was just not an option and I decided to find myself a position with a company closer to home. I was not so young anymore. It had been years since I last had to interview for employment. I dusted off my computer and updated my résumé. It would be hard. It would mean starting over, most likely with a pay cut. Nonetheless, I would do it. I decided that all things happened for a reason. The timing of it all was not the best, but I could handle it. I was just going to go out there and find another job . . . and I did.

Work was completely separate from home. Work was good. Home was not. I was another entirely different person at home. I was a sad, lonely and confused person who seemed to be always on a mission to find answers, when none could be found. It seemed I was always trying to pull myself up by my own bootstraps. I was forever searching for any article to read which would pull everything back into perspective. I always seemed to find one that would hit the nail on the head, but always came up just short of providing me with an answer which I could accept. Then I found in my mounds of documentation "The Signs of Burnout—A Checklist for Care Givers."

There were just ten items on the list. I read each one carefully. (1) Are you curtailing visits and phone calls from close friends? (2) Have you given up hobbies or activities that you have enjoyed for years? (3) Are you developing stress-related problems such as back pain, headaches, chronic feelings of fatigue and depression? (4) Are you coming down with colds, flu and other illnesses more than usual? (5) Do you have a short temper? Do you find you are getting mad in the checkout line of the grocery store? In traffic?

With friends or family? Yes . . . Yes . . . Yes . . . Yes . . . and Yes.

(6) Do you have outbursts of anger at your loved one with Alzheimer's when he or she behaves erratically or becomes difficult? (7) Have you gained or lost weight unintentionally? (8) Do you have an unshakeable feeling of despair or pessimism? (10 ) Do you complain about lack of sleep or chronic insomnia? No . . . Yes . . . Yes . . . Yes and Yes. Were these people reading my diary? It was scary how accurate each item described my behavior. Each item except for item (6). I never had outbursts of anger toward Walter. I might have been feeling it and redirected the anger quite vocally to whoever might be innocently standing next to me, but never at Walter. A close relative once verbalized that I had developed a tongue so sharp, it could clip a hedge. Only once did they ever dare to say that to me.

Here is the thing about the check list. The book went on to state that if I answered ''Yes'' to two or more of the questions, I am probably developing burnout. If I answered ''Yes'' to three or more of the questions, that indicated the need for immediate help from friends, family and social service organizations to ease my stress. It stated that I was overtaxed, and my ability to provide quality care for myself and the person with Alzheimer's was in jeopardy. There was no special advice for anyone who had answered ''Yes'' to nine out of ten. I was feeling bad. How could this be? Dad was already safely tucked away at his new home. Everything was supposed to start getting better . . . Right?

I was losing weight and I became ill. I was losing my hair. That was intensely upsetting and I cried every day as what seemed like handfuls of hair were just falling out. I developed tremendous back pain, which kept me awake night after night. I developed severe headaches and all of my muscles ached. I was having difficulty swallowing and had started throwing up blood. I now had unexplained black and blue marks all over my body and I was scared. Then I developed a case of shingles which made my whole chest area burn like fire from the inside out. It lasted for several very long months. I had always thought that shingles was an elderly affliction. It looks like I was wrong again. I noticed that I seemed to be very sensitive to bright light and loud noises too. This was something new.

I remember seeing a commercial on TV about depression. They listed the symptoms and stated that if you were experiencing any of these symptoms for a period of two weeks, the condition may be serious and to call your doctor. "Two weeks???" I shrieked, "Two weeks??? . . . how about two freaking years?" I groped for my shoe, hurling it at high speed toward the TV. Damn . . . I missed.

I was secretly very frightened and I asked David at one particularly painful and low point, that if I were to die, what would he have to say about me in my obituary.

He laughed. He laughed for Christ sake. What a stupid question from the "Drama Queen" apparently. I asked again and was amazed that this person I had loved and lived with for twenty years did not seem to know one shred of any details about my life. He didn't even know where I was born. Hello . . . same state, same town, same hospital, same place that you were born . . . idiot. "Till death do us part" had very little meaning to me anymore.

I always found it difficult in any situation to stand up and express myself in a clear, rational manner. I had been conditioned in a way, over the past twenty years or so, not to talk about what is bothering you as it is more polite to sweep it under the carpet. I was not at ease communicating my thoughts, especially if it involved someone getting close enough to me to have a peek at my soul. I also did not come off especially well if I was angry.

I had a wee bit of a temper, you see, which could sometimes get in the way of clear communication. But for some reason, I could sit down and write. Writing allowed me to slow down and organize my thoughts. Writing allowed me to speak. Indignantly, I sat at my computer and I banged out my own obituary. I pulled my self-tribute from the printer and slapped it down in front of him. "This is the person you married," I huffed.

I was alone. I looked around to find I was truly alone and had never felt like this before. I had lost interest in the simple things that had always been so important to me. I was very proud of my Irish heritage and was closely involved with my own Dad in researching the family genealogy. For years now I would dive into the microfiche and old church records, searching for the details of each family member who had gone before me, compiling volumes of treasured information of which I was most proud. This was who I was. How could I not care about something which had meant so much to me? I had lost my spirit. I had to be put here on earth for some purpose bigger than just using up the oxygen and self-destructing.

Several years ago, I designed and built a most beautiful whimsical English country perennial garden. I worked and worked to make every detail just right, every bloom, every stone, every brick walk, and every color combination carefully orchestrated. Each spring, I wouldn't even wait for the thaw. I would be out there moving rocks and dragging mulch bags, eager with visions of even a more spectacular garden than the year before. This year I looked out at a very sad, overgrown and neglected remnant of something that was once so beautiful. It didn't mean a thing to me.

A day doesn't go by where someone isn't still singing our praises for the great job we are doing. I just shake my head. My only hope is that something good and meaningful must come from all of this. Right now, I feel tired and sick. I looked old. I wondered if I should be dialing one of those crisis hotlines. No, I can do this. I didn't want some miracle pills with big long impressive medical names and I didn't want analysis. I didn't want to talk in front of a group. I couldn't talk to friends, and I certainly wasn't about to open up to a room full of strangers. I wanted to dig deeper and find my way, in my own way and in my own time.

I remember when Mom was so sick, and we were advised to have her sign a living will. We had never wanted to discuss anything like that, and we always had the attitude that there would be plenty of time for that kind of thing later.

Mom wasn't able to leave the house at that point, and so a friend of the family, who was also an attorney, agreed to make a house call. We decided that instead of having Mom face this alone with her decisions, maybe reluctant to ask questions, that we would all sign our own living wills at the same time. It worked out well, as Mom, Dad, David and myself all had our own individual concerns and questions. We all spoke up and voiced our wishes.

We all signed our living wills as a family. I was glad to have mine spelled out and signed as well. I didn't want my final wishes and decisions left up to someone else. Now that I knew that something was very wrong with my health, I was glad that I had done it. Some people acted surprised and uncomfortable when we mentioned that we had signed them together and I'm not sure exactly why. Using the family approach worked well. We had all taken care of something very important for ourselves, and it seemed to gently take the focus away from our real dreaded mission, to carry out Mom's wishes the best way we knew how.

I mustered up the very last bit of strength and courage within myself and I did two things. First, I reluctantly called my doctor and booked an appointment. This was a hard thing for me to do, as our faithful doctor always seemed to be the bearer of bad news. Second, I made my own final arrangements. Infuriated, afraid and indignant that there would be no one who would care, I took care of my own final arrangements. I also was facing the reality that we could not rely on caring children to handle things later on for us. Some people take this for granted I think, but what would they do if they had no one? I decided that it was really not a bad thing to do, perhaps a little premature, perhaps not. I was almost fifty and not well. Either way, it was the organized approach and I felt good about it.

I even designed my stone. It was a beautiful Celtic Cross, just like the ones I found in Ireland, complete with Celtic knots and engraved in Gaelic. I chose a lovely little cemetery in the town I had grown up in and I bought and paid for my own plot. I wrote everything down. I organized all of my papers and bank accounts. I had my clothes cleaned and hung in the closet with a note and all of my final instructions. It's not what you think. I wasn't looking to do myself harm, it wasn't anything like that. I was much too fond of myself for any thoughts of that. I was sick though, and very worried. It got back to one simple basic thought. I was always anally organized and liked to do things myself. I didn't want an ounce of burden or decision to fall upon other people who did not have time.

I digress . . . It was years earlier when David and I were about to be married. The family had secretly planned a surprise shower for me and David was given one task. He had to devise a plan to get me there. One Saturday morning David announced that he was going to take me fishing. This was not my favorite thing in the world, but I was always a good sport and agreed. It was spring but it was still very cold. I put layer upon layer of old baggy clothes on. I didn't bother with makeup and took little time brushing my hair as I was pulling an oversized wool hat over the mess anyway. We made our way to the brook which was miles from home and I found my spot perched upon a slippery rock.

About an hour later, David announced it was time to go. He said we needed to drop in on his brother, since his brother lived only a short distance away. I was not feeling especially attractive in my get-up but reluctantly agreed. After all, they were going to be my new family, and they might as well see the real me. I turned to grab my tackle box, but before I knew what was happening, I began sliding off of the slippery rock and found myself up to my neck in the icy cold and muddy brook. I dragged myself to shore. My clothes were drenched and dripping and now weighed about two hundred pounds. I had mud in my shoes, my hat was gone, and my stringy drippy hair was stuck to my face.

"Okay . . . " he cheerfully announced, "let's just drop in on Ray!" You must be kidding . . . I just want to go home. I protested but he insisted. When we got to Ray's, I insisted on staying in the car, but he just kept saying "oh . . . come on . . . we're just going to say hello." "Alright, but I'm staying on the steps, I'm not ruining his carpet with my drippy self."

We went up to the door and I rang the bell. The door opened and I was greeted by a thundering "Surprise!!!!!" The flashes of cameras came from every angle. The room was filled with all of my well wishing friends and relatives. My surprise shower . . . how nice.

I turned to David and shot him daggers. This was the big plan he devised? To deliver me to my shower drenched, dirty, and dressed like a pioneer woman who was having a very, very bad day. "Not to worry," David announced, flashing me a big smile "I brought clothes!" He held out a crumpled paper bag he had been hiding under his jacket for hours. Very tricky of him. I quickly made my escape to the bathroom to get somewhat cleaned up and to get changed while he entertained the guests with the story of our adventure. I could hear the laughter.

I opened the bag to find an old rumpled striped shirt, with an equally rumpled old plaid skirt. More good news . . . shoes that didn't match. I was a prisoner in this bathroom and now I was going to have to murder the groom. I emerged to the smiles and laughter of the crowd. Obviously, my shower photos were going to have to be burned. We laughed about this story over and over again for years. Now it was just another irritating example of how he didn't give my feelings or appearance an ounce of thought. I was damned sure I was not putting him in charge of dressing me for eternity when that day came.

I thought about Mom. She had clearly told her sons that she once saw a stone marker she really loved. It was made of pink granite and it had a heart engraved on it. She wanted one just like it. I was there when she described it. I wrote it down. All heads bobbed in agreement. After she died, she got instead an entirely different one, a plain grey stone, identical to David's grandparents, same size, same shape, right down to identical font. Dad said he was not about to spend eternity under a shiny pink heart. Case closed. I always felt very bad about that. I tried to say that it wasn't important. It was just a stone after all, what did it matter? It mattered to me.

In the meantime, I had designed my own Celtic Cross. A perfect replica of my descendants' stones. It was an important symbol for me. With all of the searching and researching of my genealogy for many years, my trail often lead me to some old, overgrown and very neglected cemetery on some far away hillside in Ireland. I always found, much to my delight, a most beautiful Celtic Cross at the end of my search. I thought it was very fitting for me to have one. It was a perfect symbol of who I felt I was. I took many photos of them and brought them home so I could design my own Cross.

The Gaelic epitaph was amusing as well. Not only was it a little humorous, but it was a road map of sorts. It gave a clue as to where my relatives descended from, just in case someone was researching the family history a hundred years from now, as I had done with my great-great-grandparents. I put my detailed plans together and they were to be carefully tucked away in a box. There, I thought they would stay for many years until it was my time to meet God.

They stayed in that box for all of about five minutes as David indignantly announced "Nope . . . you'll be buried next to my Mother, and you're getting a stone just like hers. Oh . . . P.S. wooden caskets are expensive, you're getting a metal one." I guess I should have been happy that he was willing to pop for something a little better than a giant Tupperware to bury me in. I took out my plans and did it myself. Okay, so way overdone on the dramatic side, I agree. I honestly felt I did not have one family member who I could rely upon to put out a little effort when it came to my wishes. Why this was so important to me, I do not know. I only knew that it was. I was glad to have done this myself. I had done them a favor and I would never have to think about this stuff again. Despite this silent tirade of self pity, one thing was perfectly clear. I did not want to die, I wanted to live.

Years ago I had compiled a list of all the things I wanted to accomplish in my life. I had succeeded with many of the items on my list, but I still had so much more to do. I had so much more to learn. I was not going out without a fight. I wanted to win, but in case I didn't, I would be prepared and take care of some details myself. I had watched with sadness and helplessness at the declining health, and deaths of other family members. I became aware of the great blessings of life. Life was a gift, not to be taken for granted. Our existence was not a mere random blip in the whole scheme of things. Each one of us was here for a purpose. Like a giant tapestry, each of us a fiber touching all those around us.

We must take the time be kind to each other. Our actions were not only affecting ourselves, but instead affecting every one whose lives we touched. It was our responsibility to be aware of this incredible ability we each had within ourselves to make things better if we chose to. We each had a destiny to fulfill, but we are free spirits as well. I once heard a speaker express my thoughts completely . . . I did not believe that I was a human being having spiritual experiences, I believed that I was a spiritual being having human experiences. I spent a lot of time thinking about that one very important thought. That carried some very large responsibilities when it came to looking at the bigger picture in life. In the meantime, I felt that those most close to me were screwing with my tapestry.

The doctor gave me an exam and did a full workup with blood tests to rule out the major critical illnesses. He was very concerned about the weight loss and the black and blue marks on my body, and gently asked me to tell him what was going on. I broke down and proceeded to spill out the events of the preceding years. God, it sounded almost shocking to hear myself saying all of these things out loud. He listened quietly for a long time and was very compassionate. He explained how stress can do very bad things to our bodies, especially long periods of continued stress. I remembered Maggie once more. I knew Maggie had once suffered physically as well as emotionally as she tried to find her way. I was determined to find a different end. I could and I would find my way through this.

I confided to him that I had been self-medicating with over the counter back pain remedies to help with the chronic pain. He explained that those were for short-term relief only, but that they contained very high dosages of aspirin-like ingredients which were breaking down my red blood cells and were causing bleeding, thus the black and blue marks and stomach pains and the vomiting of blood. I felt a rush of relief as this could be fixed. He sent me to a chiropractor to have a look at my back. I could no longer sit or stand or function without severe pain. I could barely climb up on to the table. She looked at my twisted spine and started to discuss some preliminary possibilities when the word "Scoliosis" fell from her lips.

I began to cry. She was used to seeing all kinds of things on a daily basis, and the words just rolled off of her lips with ease. I was not prepared to hear a nonchalant preliminary diagnosis. Upon further examination, she determined that the severe long-term stress effect had caused my muscles to contract so badly, that the muscles had actually pulled my vertebrae out of alignment causing the crippling pain. I felt another rush of relief . . . this too could be fixed . . . I think. I had done all of these terrible things to myself by the way I was handling, or should I say not handling my stress. Always a very healthy woman, this came as a rude awakening to me. I was harming myself and I needed to change my behavior quickly. It was very upsetting to me that I had completely neglected my poor body. It was screaming out for a little care.

A friend told me that if I ever needed a quiet place to sort things out, I could stay at a vacant apartment she owned for a few weeks before her new tenants moved in. David and my family were upset and even angry when I suggested it. They told me I couldn't just run away from my problems. I decided that I jolly well could. I could just pack up a few things and get the hell out of my surroundings for a while. I was starting to un-love those I had loved for years. I needed to gain perspective by separating myself from the whole situation. I packed my things, and left. I went to work each day as if nothing were wrong. It seems I had mastered this ability to separate my personal life from my professional life very well. I really enjoyed my work with the new company. I could be a thinking and productive person, a person who succeeded, and I really liked that person.

I stayed away from Dad too. As much as I wanted to see him, I didn't go. Every time I would visit him in the past, I would spend many hours rehashing and evaluating the events of our visit and just didn't want to subject myself to that for awhile. At night after work, I would drive to my new temporary home. It was quiet, and had no phone. I enjoyed the sound of no noise, just peace. I prepared a little supper for myself each night. I would write. I read or watched a little TV and went to bed. It was a different way of life for me, a simple existence. I didn't have to take care of anyone except for myself. I discovered that not only could I survive by myself, I could do it well. I was appreciating and even loving the skin that I was in.

My two week sabbatical ended and it was time to face the family. They were not especially impressed with my decisions of late, but that was just too bad. I rather enjoyed feeling better about myself. I needed to reconnect somehow with that person I was. An elderly relative whom I had first met only a few years ago, who also happened to be a nun, made an observation about me that I will carry with me for the rest of my life. We met at a family reunion for the first time in Ireland and had spent several days together. She studied me for a long time before she decided that she would tell me that I had a very old soul but a very young spirit.

What an interesting thing to say to someone you hardly knew. I had never given any of that much thought, thinking the whole soul-spirit thing was pretty much the same thing.

I decided she was correct. I had a deep reverence and respect for those who had gone before me, and yet a zest for life which made me dance as if no one was watching. A joyful spirit, that was me. Where did I go? Gotta get that back. I really liked that person.

My uneventful homecoming . . . It appeared that my cat hadn't missed me all that much. Patrick gave me a disinterested yawn and went and sat by his empty food dish. Some things never change. Some things do . . . David had called his brother Ray and asked for help with Dad's LLC and commercial property. His brother willingly and immediately agreed to take over the books and this part of the nightmare. That was great. Dad's house was now empty and the brothers hired a cleaning company to scour it from top to bottom. That was great. With the yard groomed, it looked nice and we had it appraised.

One final walk-though of the old place and the house was sold to an adjoining land owner who had been interested in acquiring it for some time, so that made our lives easier. In his garden across the street, Dad's raspberry bushes were now overgrown and dead. For years, he had taken so much pride in caring for them. It seemed somehow symbolic that now they were gone. Jake went to live at his new home with Ray and his kids. The big black Buick was sold. Now at least, one or two, maybe three more hurdles were jumped, and some funds were available to keep Dad going for a couple of years, anyway. Amen.

# XV
# New Friends

You know what they say, "God never closes a door without opening a window." This is one example of those unexpected blessings. I am loving this part of the journey. Dad's tapestry was growing as he was touching lives in his new home. I pretty much assumed that Dad would be placed in the facility to quietly wait out his days, and his story would fade until the end. I never expected or gave a thought to those he would meet along the way this far into his journey, and these wonderful people were now enriching my life as well. Each one, a very important part of the beautiful tapestry. Dad had developed a special rapport with some of the residents in his wing as he continued on his journey, and they were about to become my friends as well.

There was Edward, a younger man who had been diagnosed with Alzheimer's in his early fifties but was now in the advanced stages. His walls were covered with photos of his life and his journeys around the world. A once vibrant and successful businessman who now was barely able to communicate. He moved about very slowly, every action and turn of his head was done in slow motion. He would smile when you called him by name, but it would take a while before his slow moving eyes would eventually come to rest upon your face. Edward was always very neatly dressed and he was fascinated with his own shoes. Often stopping in the hall to bend down and touch them. He seemed to study them. I wondered what he was thinking. Whatever it was, I knew it was not just a random repetitive act. There was a reason.

His photos of his travels and adventures were impressive, but his greatest success in life most surely was the love of his family. His wife Elizabeth was an inspiration. She cared for him deeply. She was the first one to come over and comfort us when we would appear lost and upset with our initial visits with Dad. She told us that it was going to be okay and that he would be well taken care of. She hugged me and she didn't even know me. That small gesture meant everything.

She could be found at her husband's side, night or day, and she cared for the other residents as well. She was first in line to volunteer putting together resident activities and she liked Dad. I felt as though she was keeping a special eye on him. Elizabeth always greeted us with a smile and offered a small update on Dad's latest activities. She was tiny yet very strong, committed and truly sweet. I could learn a lot from her example. Her story was one of true love. Edward, I decided, was a lucky man.

There was Arthur, another gentleman in his early seventies. His shadow box was empty so I could only wonder about his life and family. It bothered me that the box was just hanging there completely empty outside his door. What I did know was that he was special. His soft and kind mannerisms reminded me of Dad. I would call him by name and his face would light up. He would speak in broken thought patterns, but his eyes and personality spoke volumes. He was an interesting man with an interesting story, I was sure of that. He seemed comfortable in his surroundings and never appeared agitated. He should have been retired in his old Victorian house, a grandpa sitting in his great big favorite chair with all of his grandchildren gathered around him.

When I think of Arthur, I think of a warm Norman Rockwell holiday drawing. That's where he should have ended up, in a Norman Rockwell drawing to live out his remaining years, passing down stories of the old days, chewing on his old worn out pipe, and cherishing his family life in quiet comfort. I always enjoyed seeing him. He was a kind soul. If he wasn't in the community area, I found myself seeking him out just to say hello. It wasn't too long before Arthur was gone. I don't know what became of him, as there are strict rules regarding patient confidentiality so the staff is very limited when it comes to giving details, but I will never forget him.

There was Louis, a tough old guy who barked out gruff encoded dialog. He intimidated some of the other residents, including Dad. He could always be found in the community living room, eyes fixed to the television, arms crossed, and always in the same chair. His chair, and the other residents respected that. I felt he had a distrust for everyone. I suspect he would have made a great staff sergeant, yes . . . surely an old military man. I ventured down the hall to give his shadow box a look.

Louis was instead a farmer and I smiled at my miscalculation. His box was filled with memories of a much younger man, always toiling away with various farm equipment. The camera never seemed to catch him with a smile. It did catch his devotion to hard work and his pride in what he had accomplished. He had high standards and things needed to be done his way. That much was clear. A tough man his whole life. I liked this man. I made my way back down the hall and sat down next to him. "Hi Louis . . . . I'll bet you had a beautiful farm," I said. His gaze slowly moved from the TV to my face and he studied me in silence for some time. With each visit, I would always stop to say hello to Louis.

Each time Louis would silently study me. Eventually the day came when I said my usual "Hello, Louis" but this time I detected a small trace of a smile cross his lips. I jumped when he barked out a loud, abrupt "Hello." I chuckled to myself as I wondered what I must have looked like when I jumped. I smiled back at him. Louis's progression came in the form of agitation and we began witnessing his increased argumentative and physical outbursts with the staff. The day came when Louis was no longer there. His shadow box was empty and his room cleaned. Every last trace of Louis had vanished.

Stella was an interesting woman. She was wheelchair bound and always clutched a ragged doll. She would sit for hours stroking the doll's matted hair and rocking it back and forth. She would only speak in long, loud and cryptic rambling. She was an irritation to the other residents as she would carry on day and night. In the dining room, she was placed at a table by herself in the corner. I could not pick up on any of her personality traits. She was in her final stages. She was not a happy woman and did not appear to respond to anyone. Her shadow box clearly showed that her religion and her family were her priorities, yet I never saw her with a visitor. I felt she was all alone in her world just waiting for God.

Months after meeting Stella, we were in the dining room having dinner with Dad and something amazing happened. The aide delivered Stella her dessert, and to everyone's surprise, Stella clearly responded, "Thank you very much. The dinner was delicious." We all looked around wondering where that voice came from. The aide saw our surprised looks and told us that every once in a while, just for a fleeting rare moment, Stella comes back to us and speaks as clear as day. Almost as soon as it comes, it goes again. That was the one and only moment I ever really met Stella.

Months later I noticed Stella was gone. Another resident saw me peeking in her room and told me that the men came in that night and "put a black tablecloth on her." The next day, I saw her obituary. There was her picture. A beautiful young woman and her life story. Stella had the same birthday as me, but she had been born forty-three years earlier. She was an avid photographer. I found that part of her story to be most amazing. There was no clue of that captured in her shadow box. She was also deeply religious, was a devoted wife, mother, grandmother and great-grandmother.

She was an accomplished seamstress and she played the piano. Stella was a wonderful human being as well. The tribute listed her work with many volunteer organizations over the years. She had helped with the war effort by working at an old military air strip which has long since become our local commercial airport. She had also been a teacher for many years. Clearly, Stella was a nice woman who had helped people her whole life. The obituary went on to say that Stella was predeceased by an infant daughter.

I thought about the Stella I knew. It had appeared to me that all of her cherished memories from her life had faded completely away, yet, somewhere deep inside of her, she was showing us her deep love for her infant daughter. Right to the end, when nothing else seemed to make sense, she continued to clutch her doll, gently holding it and stroking its matted hair, rocking it gently back and forth. I felt comforted to know that she was now reunited with her little girl. She had broken free from her own sadness, from her own tragic loop.

Tilly was a pip. I love Tilly. She sat at Dad's table during meal time and always kept the ball rolling. In her eighties, she had the ability to make everyone dive out of her path for fear of being run over by her trademark walker. She could wheel that thing around like it was nobody's business. I asked her if "Tilly" was short for "Matilda" but she didn't know. Her hair was always in a wild mess. The buttons on her sweater were never quite matched up to the right button holes. I once asked her if she needed a little help getting her buttons straightened out. "Oh no dear, I already did that myself," she replied. Tilly loved to smile, the old false teeth always dropping out, usually on her plate during dinner. We became accustomed to this quickly, and often helped her fish them out.

In her younger years, she was a fiery redhead, and she often told me so. She was now an avid NASCAR fan of all things and never missed a weekend race, unless she forgot. Most of the time she forgot. Her grandchildren called her "NASCAR Nana." She talked about the races and how she had to cheer for "Her Boys." I smiled as I quipped "Atta Girl Tilly!" Little did she know, we had something in common. She frequently invited me to her room to show me their pictures. She thought that Dale Earnhardt Jr. was pretty good, but she thought his father was the cat's pajamas. She spoke of him in the present tense and I had a feeling she didn't realize he had died in a crash several years earlier.

Her warm personality shone through with a brilliance. Tilly would show us the facility grounds and describe in great detail how she planted each and every plant in the beautiful gardens. Her labors took her at least ten years, she said. She described her meticulous planning and planting, over and over again. It didn't matter to me that the facility was only a few years old and that she had only been there a little longer than Dad. I always told her she did a wonderful job and she would beam with pride.

My favorite image of Tilly became engraved permanently in my mind one cold winter night. The facility hosted many activities which included dances complete with small brass bands playing the "oldies." I would watch with amazement as even the most advanced residents who no longer seemed to respond at all, would suddenly come to life with the sounds of Glenn Miller. Tilly was no exception. Her feet would start tapping and she began bouncing in her seat.

David was always a great sport and asked her to dance. Tilly's eyes burned with excitement. She flung her walker aside and the next thing you know, her arms and legs were flailing out of control in all directions as she danced. The staff was calling out to David to hold on to her. Everyone watched with delight. Tilly was grinning from ear to ear. David looked frightened, afraid of being kicked no doubt, or perhaps afraid those teeth were going to fly across the dance floor.

I laughed as a vision of my favorite episode of *Seinfeld* popped into my head. Any loyal viewer would surely remember the "Elaine Dance" episode. At a posh corporate affair, the music started, and a very proper and professional Elaine suddenly began to dance, shocking the stuffy crowd with her outrageous, most uncoordinated flailing of limbs. The crowd went silent, Elaine totally unaware of her frightening display, convinced she must be really great if all of these co-workers stopped what they were doing to watch her. Whispers and looks followed at work the next day, Elaine still unaware of the embarrassing scene she had created with her "talent."

That was certainly Tilly to a tee. The floor cleared as the crowd watched. The staff members were all holding their breath. The song ended and a sweaty and very relieved David escorted her back to her seat. No limbs broken, thank God. He politely thanked her for the dance. She nonchalantly told him that he was out of step. Tilly was a happy soul. Her shadow box showed that she loved to travel. It was packed with photos of her life's adventures. Young or old, the images of Tilly's face were always shining with a huge smile. I am thinking I would like to become just like Tilly when I get old.

Then there was Henry. Henry reminded me of a cartoon character, in a way, like Mr. Magoo. In his eighties, a short, slight yet impeccably groomed smiley-type character who was always on a mission. He squinted and was always bumping into things. He fancied himself a ladies man, always sporting a clean white pressed shirt and bow tie. He was always winking at the girls and I was forever telling him that I needed to keep my eye on him. He would beam and chuckle. Henry was stuck in a loop too. He was constantly adding numbers and making lists.

He had very important work and deadlines that he was always fretting over. Numbers . . . numbers . . . recalculating, more lists, lots of stress. We decided he must have been an accountant or auditor. Henry was a man of order and method. He could talk for hours, and often did, about things not adding up. He had solutions and a plan, a big plan for when he got out of here. He was very vocal about how the whole system was corrupt, yet we could never quite pin down what he was talking about.

Henry was usually up to something and always very sure about himself. I'm glad that he didn't realize that sometimes his pants were on inside out, the inside white lining and pockets dangling on the outside like sails. Sometimes the pants were missing all together, but he was still sporting the crisp white shirt and bow tie. Then one day he sadly confided in us. He told us he had a secret. He told us that everyone he knew was dead. Everyone except for two people, he said. He told us that he talks to God.

God was trying to tell Henry something very important but he couldn't quite understand what God was saying. Henry said he had been listening very hard, but he can't quite hear him yet. It seems, to be honest, I feel the same way sometimes. "Henry, I know exactly what you are saying," I told him. His son once told me that Henry was a brilliant engineer. He had designed important parts for military planes, parachutes and other vital components during the war effort. He held a top position with a very large aircraft company for many years up until his retirement.

Last but not least was my very special friend, Andrew. Andrew was a very quiet, small wisp of a man, his baggy pants being held up with his oversized belt like a drawstring. Andrew immediately became attached to Dad. He would follow Dad everywhere, up and down the halls right on his heels. Dad would politely tell him that he didn't need to do that, but Andrew just smiled as he continued anyway. He viewed Dad as the leader. Pretty soon, Dad was leading the parade.

Other residents were falling in line behind Andrew, everyone shuffling along in a tidy line. Dad would shrug and roll his eyes. Andrew's shadow box displayed his high school yearbook photo with the printed description of him as a quiet, studious and nice young man. "A man of few words" it read. I think he had some kind of a clock repair business too. Maybe it was just a hobby.

I would always give Andrew a big giant "Helloooo" and he would beam. His big giant smile would reveal a lone, single tooth just barely dangling down. His eyes would twinkle. He would always look at me and say "You're beautiful!" I would smile and say "You're beautiful too, Andrew!" He liked that. He would pause for a moment, turn and shuffle away. No matter how old you get, it's nice when someone tells you you're beautiful. I am no exception. It didn't matter that he was probably about ninety years old, suffering from Alzheimer's and had cataracts, I still appreciated him saying so. I would always walk away feeling a little better about myself.

One day we crossed paths in the hall and Andrew gave me my usual "You're beautiful" compliment. I smiled and cheerfully continued on my way. He always brightened up my day and that day I felt beautiful! A few moments later, I heard Andrew's far away voice again . . . . "You're beautiful." I turned around to see Andrew standing in the corner. He was talking to the fire extinguisher. Wow . . . that smacked my ego right back down to size. I had a good laugh with myself just the same. It was just so funny. The cruel irony of it all.

The alarm clock went off and I crawled out of bed. I was mentally organizing all the things I had to do at work that day. I stirred my coffee and opened the paper. There was a picture of a very young Andrew in the obituaries. He had died at the age of eighty-seven. What a handsome young man, a veteran, having served with the U.S. Air Force in World War II while stationed somewhere in England. He attended Harvard University and was an Attorney and Vice President for a large company for many years. Andrew loved baseball and was a Red Sox fan. His hobbies were repairing antique clocks and woodworking. He was survived by his wife and three daughters. To me . . . he was just Andrew. Another one of my special friends who found their way into my heart. These very sweet souls would never know that they were helping me heal.

The aides told me about a woman named Emma. A newer resident in Dad's house. She had her big green eyes set on Dad. They would eat together and take walks together. She spoke very softly and it was very hard for her to put her thoughts together. Dad was very patient with her and would softly ask her to explain again. I thought that she resembled Mom. She was very attractive, beautiful hair and clothes. She carefully assembled all of her mounds of jewelry, layer upon layer as she wore it all at once. The staff thought that the two of them just might be able to help each other and Emma was all for it. She would light up when she saw Walter, and we immediately liked her. She was so quiet and sweet, never a harsh word, a real lady. One day we arrived to find Emma grinding her teeth, making huffing noises, very agitated and looking out the window. Trouble in paradise. The aides gave us wide-eyed looks.

# XVI

## "Anne & Paul"
## aka
## "Eleanor & Walter"

It seems that there was a new woman zooming in on Emma's turf. Her name was Eleanor. Eleanor was the new resident and she and Walter made an immediate connection. I tried to figure it out. Eleanor had to be at least ten years older than Walter, putting her at age eighty-six-ish. She was sweet and frail now. What was interesting to me is that she resembled Grandma, Walter's mother. Not so much with her looks, it was more her lady-like mannerisms. I knew that she was very smart, in more ways than one. She also reminded me of Grandma because she was a woman way ahead of her time.

Years ago, in a man's world, Eleanor was out there pioneering as a designer. Graduating in 1946 with a Bachelor of Fine Arts from the Rhode Island School of Design. Her stories were very interesting and informative. She had traveled all over the world and gave detailed accounts of her adventures. Not your common type of conversation you hear in this place. Eleanor smelled of roses . . . not the typical "eau d' urine" I had become accustomed to in this place.

Her career was her life and she never married. Her only relative was her devoted nephew. Her only brother had passed away a few years before. Eleanor had beautiful eyes, and I imagined her as a beautiful and spunky young woman.

Walter and Eleanor quickly became inseparable. They strolled the halls, hand in hand. They ate together and Eleanor was even getting Dad to join in on all of the community room activities. Dad had stopped packing his clothes to leave again and he was happy. Eleanor's condition was far less progressed than Walter's, and Eleanor seemed to take him under her wing. Eleanor would become confused at times, but seemed to bounce back and she could continue where she left off. The staff approved of this match now too. She was really getting Walter to join in.

Everyone was happy. Everyone, that is except for Emma. This normally quiet as a mouse little lady was now barking at Walter. "Where have you been??" boomed out of that little body whenever she would catch sight of Walter. Walter would react confused and startled. He was not used to yelling. Emma would cast evil glares in Eleanor's direction, and she didn't have much use for us either. When Walter would leave his room, Emma would go in and leave her belongings there on his bed. Her purse, her clothes, things like that.

I don't think Walter really understood what was going on. Actually, I am more than sure that Walter did not understand. Emma was nothing more than a faded confused memory. His life was quickly revolving around Eleanor. For my part, I thought it was sweet. I liked her and I was stepping back. This was good. He was safe. I was feeling better. I was sleeping again and gaining back some weight. Life had a way of figuring itself out.

So far it all seemed quite innocent, except for the hurting Emma part. An interesting thing was taking place though, which I was not comfortable with. Eleanor had a boyfriend many years ago and his name was Paul. I'm thinking that Paul was the love of her life. It wasn't long before she stopped calling Walter by his name and began calling him Paul. That was okay, I guess as Dad was now calling her "Anne" or "Mom" as he used to call Anne.

We would come for a visit and he would excitedly exclaim, "Let's go find Mom!" It seems that his mind had simply replaced fifty years of memories of Anne with Eleanor. There was a framed picture of Mom in his room, and we asked him once who it was. "That's Mom, let's go find Mom, she's right down the hall . . . there she is, let's go see Mom." We looked down the hall and there was Eleanor, smiling from ear to ear and giving us all a big wave. We were always confused but confident that we would eventually figure it all out.

# XVII

## "Make Sure You Knock. . . . I Said. . . . Make Sure You Knock"

We arrived one day as usual and began looking for Dad. He was nowhere to be found. We searched all of the usual places but still no sign of him. We asked the head nurse if she had seen him, and she smiled. "You'll probably find him in Eleanor's room . . . but make sure you knock . . . I said make sure you knock." The two of us stood there like two adult dummies, mouths hanging open. "I'm not going in . . . you go in," I said. David said, "I'm not going in." Hello . . . we're both still standing here, afraid to move. An aide spotted us and said she would go in. After a few minutes, smiling Dad and smiling Eleanor emerged from the room.

We all went for a walk. Dad was a little irritated with the staff. It seems that they wouldn't allow him to sleep with his wife. He said they were always telling him he must go back to his own room. He would gravitate between thinking she was his wife, to repeatedly asking her to marry him. She always declined. She would tell him that she was "Much too young to get married!" He had devised an intricate plan which involved us bringing over the big black Buick and parking it in the bushes. He took us over to the window and pointed right to the spot where we needed to park.

He told us that he was taking Mom away from this place and back to their home. If we wouldn't do that for him, maybe we could just get the Buick over here for a little while, say, for a few hours . . . . Whatever did he mean by that? Who were we anyway, Bonnie and Clyde driving the getaway car? I was pretty sure I was not about to back seat drive Dad on this adventure. Good Heavens . . . . I didn't find this one in my pile of books, web sites and easy reference guides.

A few weeks later, we got "The Call." It was like being hauled into the Principal's office only worse, much, much worse. David and his brother Raymond, Eleanor's nephew, social workers and the facility administrator just for good measure met behind closed doors.

They all needed to come to an agreement. The Staff had dealt with resident romances before, but it was important that the families involved all agreed that it was not inappropriate. Were we supposed to sign a permission slip for Dad to have sex, or what? Were they just holding hands and kissing each other once in a while? What??? Wait, don't tell me, I really, really don't want to know. There was nothing better than a room full of red-faced adults discussing their parent figures' love lives.

I personally did not object to whatever they were doing, as long as no one was getting hurt. Eleanor's nephew was not on board and I could certainly understand his feelings. I still wasn't actually sure what they were doing. I did not want that vision forever imbedded in my brain. If it were my aunt or mother, I might have viewed this, whatever it was, as a dreadful violation. They both had Alzheimer's for God sake. They were calling each other by the wrong names, but you know what? They both found happiness in their world as they know it. Maybe we should leave them alone. I don't know.

How would we know if either one of them was getting hurt? I don't know. I'm certainly the last person in the world who needed to voice an opinion. The supervisor assured us all that they would be watched carefully. Great . . . . I'll be sure to sit by the phone waiting for an update. I only know one thing. Wherever Mom is right now, heaven or elsewhere, right now I'm pretty sure she is pissed. Walter and Eleanor's romance was to continue for only a short while longer. Was this good or was this bad? I don't know! I'm sure the experts have the answers. Where's the Tylenol?

# XVIII
# Eleanor . . . Eleanor Who???

We got an upsetting phone call late one night. It was the nurse from the facility saying that Dad was all upset and confused. She handed the phone to him, and she was right. Something was dreadfully wrong and he couldn't communicate it. We got dressed and sped off. We found Dad sitting on his bed all confused and tortured. He was crying. We went to Eleanor's room and she wasn't there. Her belongings were all there but she was gone. We asked the nurse what had happened to Eleanor and I could see by the look on her face that she wanted to explain, but she was bound by patient confidentiality.

We calmed Dad down and tried to get some information from him. He didn't know what was wrong. He only knew something had happened, something bad had happened. We asked if it was about Eleanor. He didn't know who we were talking about. David said "Your lady friend, Dad, is it about your lady friend?" Dad didn't know. "Mom . . . " David said, "is it about Mom?" Dad didn't know. He wasn't sure why he had the nurse call us. He said everything was fine. We tucked him in and went home. Our minds were filled with all kinds of horrible scenarios which must have happened. Where was Eleanor? Had she died or had her family walked in on something, decided enough was enough and pulled her out of there . . . but her belongings were still in her room, her shadow box intact.

The next day we returned. This time the day nurse approached us. She said that they couldn't talk to us about Eleanor until she had the family's permission. She had called them earlier that day and they said she could explain the details to us. It seems that on the previous day, Eleanor's nephew had picked her up to take her to a doctor's appointment. She had a bad fall in the parking lot, breaking her hip and her arm. I had a momentary vision of the ghost of Anne sticking her foot out in front of poor, frail Eleanor.

She was taken to the hospital and they were not sure when she would be returning, if at all. Eleanor's nephew had made a special trip back to the facility to tell Dad that night, but Walter just didn't understand. Within a few hours Dad had worked himself into a terrible state but he didn't know why. We sat Dad down and slowly explained what had happened. He seemed surprised, but acted as if we were talking about a stranger. A week later, the staff told us that Dad had been wandering the halls looking for her and visiting her room, but in a quiet and confused way. He never asked questions. It was as if he knew something was wrong, or different, but he just didn't seem to know what it was.

We went to the hospital to visit Eleanor. She was happy to see us and asked questions about Dad. She was worried about him. We could see she was in a lot of pain and very uncomfortable in her traction apparatus. A few weeks later she was moved to a local nursing home. We decided to take Dad to visit her. We spiffed him up and bought flowers for him to give to her. He was very agreeable but confused as to who she was. All the way there we were coaching him on her name and who she was, rehearsing how he would give her the flowers.

We got there and were told that her nephew had taken her to visit a friend. We left and brought Dad back to his home. When we arrived back, the staff told us that Eleanor's nephew had brought her to see Dad and they had just left! We piled back into the car, flowers in hand and drove back to the nursing home, still coaching Dad all the way. We were trying too hard to help make everything work out right. I wasn't even sure what "working out right" was. Our hearts were always in the right place, but we were just never quite on the right track. Right train . . . wrong track. None of this mattered. The important thing was to get Dad to the nursing home to visit Eleanor.

We were a little nervous that Dad might let on that he didn't know her and hurt her feelings. Dad was the greatest. We found her room and pointed Dad in the right direction. He produced a giant smile and a hearty "hello." He bent down and kissed her. He proudly displayed the flowers he brought her, telling her he had picked them out just for her because he knew she would like them. She was so happy. We were amazed as he didn't skip a beat. No wonder we can never figure out what is going on. Dad was just so convincing. On the way home, we asked Dad some questions about where we had just been. He didn't know . . . Eleanor who???

By now Emma (you remember scorned Emma) was cheerful, smiling and practically skipping about the place. She was fully aware that something dreadful had happened to Eleanor. Of that, I am sure. She still had her eyes on Dad, but he didn't even notice her. She began to sulk about the place and eventually her family moved her to a different facility. Several months went by before Eleanor returned. We were all delighted, but things were much different. She was now attached to a walker and the family had hired a private duty nurse to watch her every move.

Dad didn't acknowledge her as "Mom" anymore, and although she continued to dote on him, he politely treated her more like a stranger. She was still spending every minute she could helping him and guiding him on what to do next, but it was different. The facility held an outdoor picnic that July, complete with a brass band playing away in the gazebo. Eleanor sat quietly with her private duty nurse at a table on the opposite side of the grounds.

One night we got a call from Eleanor's nephew. He told us that they were most likely moving her to another facility after the holidays. They were worried about how this would affect Dad. He said the new facility would give her a more "private" environment with her own living room. It was more like a small apartment. He was very considerate, caring and wise. We deduced that Eleanor had her hands full taking care of Dad. Everyone could see that at times, he was becoming more and more dependant on her for his every move.

At other times, she was a stranger to him. She was too old and tired to keep up the regime of care giver. We understood of course, and were grateful for the brief time their lives had come together. We arrived on Christmas Eve with a lovely gift basket for Eleanor. We brought another gift for her that was going to be from Dad. We were too late. Her room was empty and she was gone. The smell of roses had vanished. Dad didn't seem to notice her absence, and he never mentioned her again.

# XIX

# Happy New Year

Dad has been here now for over a year and a half. A lot has happened. I look in the mirror and see an old person looking back at me. Alzheimer's has been in the news a lot lately, especially with the recent death of Ronald Reagan. He and his family struggled for twenty years. How did they ever make it through twenty years? I watched the funeral on TV and smiled quietly as his children gave beautiful eulogies. They talked about the lessons their Dad taught them as they were growing up. They didn't focus on the President or on the movie star, they talked about their Dad. Young Ron told a simple story which reminded me of a story David told me about his Dad.

Walter's three boys were little then. Dad went out into the backyard and was showing them the proper use of a homemade slingshot. He was very careful to teach them never to harm an animal or another human being. He had fashioned this slingshot with a stick and the elastic from an old pair of underpants. The three boys hung on his every word. Dad was always their hero. He demonstrated how to hold the thing, picking up a small stone and randomly fired it into the tree as he spoke sternly yet gently about safety.

A second later a poofffff-thud sound could be heard and they all stood speechless as a small bird fell from the tree dead to the ground. Dad was so upset at what he had just done that he broke the slingshot into tiny pieces and commanded his young sons to never . . . ever . . . do that. He was so angry with himself for harming that creature, and for doing that in front of his kids. Dad was the kind of man you would instead find up on a ladder in a tree, replacing little fallen baby birds to their nest. That was Dad.

Walter hasn't known me since Thanksgiving. He liked me though because I was that nice lady who always brought him chocolates. I wasn't sad. I was prepared for this. Okay . . . so maybe I was a little bit sad. Dad still loved me only he just didn't know it. The holidays came and Dad's youngest son Jackie and his family flew up from Florida. He didn't really seem to know them either although he was still the master of keeping the conversation ball rolling. He was still calling David by name and for that, I was grateful. Old friends would visit and continue to report back to us that he was "perfect," "remembering the old days in perfect detail." Blah . . . Blah . . . Blah . . .

We stopped for a moment to look at Dad's shadow box. He didn't recognize any of our faces anymore, not even Anne in their wedding photo. We knew he really had no idea about the faces in his shadow box, but we always stopped to look at it anyway, hoping for just a little glimmer of recognition. He studied it for a moment and then pointed to the photo of his parents. "That's Mom and Pop," he said. He was right. My jaw dropped as I watched his face studying the other photos. "Was that my old Navy ship?" Right again. Every other smiling face in the box were strangers. We were now giving clues in a desperate effort to spark his memory. I took the shadow box off the wall and home for repairs. Some of the old photos were beginning to fade and curl. It needed a little care.

Dad seemed to be retreating more and more from life and into his own little world. He never mentioned going home anymore. I was glad that his memories of his home had faded. What a strange thing for me to say. His little bits of memories that came and went when Walter first arrived at the facility only served as torture for him. This was somehow better. He now appears to have graduated to the middle or moderate phase. He wanders the halls and he has difficulty sleeping. He was tired and cold all of the time. He was becoming less sociable and less aware of the feelings of others. He needed help in making all decisions, and he needed assistance with bathing, grooming and dressing. Thank God we have still escaped the drastic personality changes, the sudden mood shifts, the worry and fearfulness. Walter was changing . . . . But he was still so very kind.

David took him to his doctor for a physical. He was losing weight but otherwise still very healthy for a man his age. His personal habits were changing and they now had him in "Daddy Diapers." One day Walter told David that he didn't think he was getting any better. His doctor agreed with the facility's most current evaluation. Dad's condition was reassessed from mild to moderate. The next classification would be severe or advanced. The newer residents were definitely in better shape than Dad. I was still busy thanking God that his personality had not changed. That was something I could always be sure of, his personality would never change. He was still the same sweet man he always was and I was confident that we had escaped this one dreadful trademark symptom of the disease.

We attended seminars which focused on the various drugs available in the handling of Alzheimer's Disease. The seminars were presented by the FDA, right at the facility. They were interesting and we learned that four million people in the U.S. have Alzheimer's. If you add to this the number of family members whose lives were now affected by their loved one who is suffering, the number of people affected is now staggering. Yes . . . all of this is interesting, but just how is any of this going to help Walter? The wall was covered with charts and graphs. Hmmmm . . . all very interesting. Statistics show this . . . statistics show that.

The FDA explained how the process could be slowed for the short term with some people, but eventually their decline would bring them to the same level in the long run. No cures and none of the news was promising at this point but we already knew that. At best, the drugs may sustain a better quality of life for him in the short term. Statistics show improvements may be possible for cognitive memory. The side effects . . . does this really matter? A lot of those web sites I used to scour would start off with sad testimonials. A sad family member would re-live the anguish of their declining loved one, really working on the readers' emotions. Inevitably, they would get to the point. They were advertisements for the drug companies.

The old skipping record is now thankfully a forever and forgotten broken record. Walter has escaped from his "how did I end up in this place" loop. He never ever talks about it anymore. It has been a long journey for him so far and his face is beginning to show it. He doesn't seem to be worried about anything but he looks very tired. He looks old to me too. He has begun to urinate in his radiator at the far end of his room. No matter how they barricade the radiator below his window, he continues with this new form of behavior. They have taped big signs on his bathroom door which read "TOILET" and they moved his large dresser in front of the window. Nothing seems to work. He moves the furniture and continues with this new thing. The staff was baffled.

It was David who came up with the answer to why it was happening. At Mom and Dad's old home, they had a very small and narrow bathroom. You had to practically turn sideways to maneuver past the sink and tub and make your way toward the window. The window was positioned over the toilet. This had to be what Dad was thinking. He was thinking about or subconsciously associated this area of his room with his old house and he remembered he had to head toward the window. Good job, David.

We still haven't figured out how to correct this but at least we are understanding the method to his madness. Dad is perplexed about the whole thing. He would never do something like that. He also doesn't know what to do with the toothpaste these days. He is using his toothbrush to comb his hair. Now he is washing his hands in the toilet. The money is beginning to dwindle. The features of his face are fading and his shoes are on the wrong feet again.

# XX
# Get Outa My Chair

I was at work when the next call came. David answered and was greeted by a stern voice. "David, we have a big problem, and this type of behavior is unacceptable!" David locked up his shop once again and drove to Dad's. This time there was real trouble. Dad had become protective of his belongings and was now a little territorial. Just outside of his door is a small sitting area decorated like a porch. Two large wicker chairs fill the small area. Each of the four houses within the facility have the identical setup. It seems that Dad had decided that these chairs were his.

He became irritated if a passer-by decided to sit in his chairs. Most would vacate when instructed, but not today. Today an elderly woman resident sat down. Dad had sternly suggested that she move along and she would not. The nurses heard the commotion from down the hall and came running. They arrived in time to witness Dad slap her and "help" her out of the chair and to her feet so she could be on her way. They said the woman was not hurt but she was very upset and crying.

The supervisor was very stern with David and that made me mad. She stated again that Walter's behavior was unacceptable and I found this to be most insulting. Of course we know this! He is not a child that we can simply stand in a corner until he learns his lesson. The man is progressing with Alzheimer's and you people are the paid professionals. What exactly were we expected to do? She insinuated that he could not stay if his behavior could not be corrected. This whole thing was a terrible blow.

This was why he was in this facility in the first place . . . . He was there because we didn't know what to do. She needed to take a good long look at her own damn brochure! The one with the daisies on the cover and the happy, smiling residents. The reassuring words of professional care, administered by a loving and caring staff, those reassuring words of encouragement as our loved one gently would pass though the stages of this terrible disease. It was crap. It was corporate marketing department crap!

David was instructed to come back for a meeting with the social worker and the geriatric psychologist. His work would just have to wait again while we paid giant dollars for psychoanalysis. Maybe he should just forget about his job altogether while he searched for another facility that would take Walter. They analyzed Dad, and he only remembers "helping the poor woman up from the chair." David's brother in Florida determined that Dad could be put in a facility down there for a fraction of the cost. The snotty supervisor backed down quickly when David told her he was looking into other options. Her tone immediately changed, no doubt due to the thought of the loss of that hefty chunk of money, more than five thousand dollars, being deposited on their door step each month so Dad could live there. "Let's not be hasty now . . . I'm sure we can come up with a solution." she said with a forced sickly-sweet tone.

Then came more analysis and observation. The solution was to put Dad on the latest drug. This will "enhance his quality of life." This combined with a sedative to "lessen his aggression" would certainly solve the problem. They had no way of figuring out what may have triggered the incident to start with. David thought for a moment and responded again with the answer. Mom and Dad had a small porch just off of their living room complete with wicker chairs. They also had two large Adirondack chairs where they spent many summer evenings side by side. These were Dad's memories and it may have explained why he reacted the way he did when a stranger would not move. It was not an excuse, it was an explanation. Good job, David.

Today was February 18th. As I tossed and turned in bed, I was listening to the loud strange noises my stomach had started making again. I looked up at the ceiling fan and calculated that Mom has been gone now for 826 days. I am very upset. Upset for the poor woman who was mistreated and upset for Dad. How many times have I lovingly spoke of Dad's unchanging kind, gentle and most wonderful personality. That was our most precious gift. Up until now, we remained untouched by this part of the progression.

He had never hit anyone in his life. He never ever would have hit a woman. He was a gentleman. This horrible disease has now violated his soul, his innermost core of goodness. I called out to Mom. I asked her to please ask God to take Dad. I couldn't watch this beautiful person turn into a mean, angry or violent person. Walter was a kind and gentle soul. That little voice from inside my head replied that it was not yet his time and we all still had more lessons to be learned, a few more miles on his journey down the road of life.

# XXI

## Seasons

"Everything has its time . . . . To everything there is a season, a time for every purpose under heaven." This is the time to dig deeper within ourselves. I felt terribly guilty for taking the cowardly approach by asking God to take him home now so it would be over and we might begin to heal. I apologized to God once again as I know in my heart that I learn a little something from Dad each time I see him. I recalled my thoughts as we started this journey, that he touched each of us as we were learning our own individual and very personal life's lessons along the way. Our own self-discovery was his special gift to each one of us, and I needed to find a way to appreciate this.

My thoughts however, now changed toward that poor woman who was slapped that day for sitting in his chair. My horror of the vision of this poor, frail, and totally innocent woman had changed. This just could not have happened as his now permanent file entries suggested. Surely she must have been evil. Evil enough to make this kind and gentle soul, this wonderful man become agitated with her. I might just have to make a trip over there myself, track her down, and issue at very least, a good strong tongue lashing or worse, just for getting Dad in trouble. Good God! What am I thinking . . . this is probably not the lesson I should be learning right now . . . I need to focus back on the love thing, and fast.

Money worries continued and talk of moving Dad to Florida again was coming up in conversation. "It's a lot cheaper down there . . . " I didn't want to hear it again. No way were we packing him up and moving him away from this environment that he called home. The comment was made that he was "an empty shell of a man." I was outraged. I told David that he needed to visit Dad and listen, and for the hundredth time . . . stop finishing his sentences. David has resumed his routine of telling Dad what he thinks he means, and as usual, Dad still agrees with everything he says. I can see that he is slipping further away, but Walter was not "an empty shell of a man."

It was a bitter cold and snowy day when the invitation arrived. The facility was hosting the Annual Snowball Ball. We were instructed to dress formally, and to bring formal clothes for Dad. We gussied ourselves up and I asked David to call in an order to the florist. I wanted a boutonniere for Walter and one for David too. We stopped to pick up the order and David smiled as he surprised me with a beautiful matching corsage which he had ordered for me. We headed off for a night of adventure. David's brother Ray and his girlfriend were coming too. That was going to be great.

We arrived to hear the sounds of Glenn Miller once more. The wonderful aroma of the buffet filled the halls. We got Dad all ready and I pinned on his white carnation. He looked dashing. I really enjoyed seeing the other residents and the staff all decked out. Feet were tapping, residents were smiling, some dancing. David loosened his tie and was fidgeting in the corner. He was scanning the room and no doubt hiding from Tilly. He was still having nightmares from their last dance together. She found him and the scene was repeated, except this time I had my video camera! This tape would be worth money someday!

A nice slow song began to play. I asked Henry to dance. He looked very dashing with his bow tie. His pants were on, right side out. As the music continued, I took him gently by the arm. We took careful baby steps, a slow motion shuffle, stopping to rest every few steps as we made our way to the dance floor. Onlookers were smiling, admiring my patience I'm sure. By the time we finally made it to the floor, the song was over and the band leader announced they were going to step it up with a lively jitterbug type number.

I looked at him with a mortified expression. "You must be joking . . . . I beg you, I am begging you to play another slow, very slow song!" I shouted out in desperation. The crowd laughed and so did the band leader. He smiled with a glint in his eye, as he too had watched my long hard journey to the dance floor with Henry. He willingly obliged and played us a lovely slow golden oldie.

Henry and I had the whole dance floor to ourselves. The crowd clapped, we both smiled and Henry bowed. We then began that long slow journey back to his chair. I watched Dad carefully that night, wondering what the view from his world was looking like these days. We danced together. He sang along to the oldies, and danced like Fred Astaire. He never stopped smiling once. The ladies were lining up to dance with him. The music . . . something about the music had such a powerful way of reaching these people. It was wonderful. Dad's old charm was really at work. He was really having fun, and could dance without missing a step. The band was packing up and Dad still wanted to continue dancing.

At one point during the night, Dad and I took a break and we were walking arm in arm down the hall. One of the nurses stopped to tell us how nice we looked all dressed up in our formal wear. The nurse asked Walter who I was. At first he introduced me as his wife, although he couldn't remember my name. Then he told her he wasn't sure just who I was. I really wanted him to say, "This is my daughter-in-law, Janet," but he just kind of stood there, puzzled and scratching his head. He seemed confused at the thought that he was being led around by someone he didn't know. Maybe there was some far away glimmer of a feeling, not so much a memory. Maybe there was a comfort level deep inside of him which still allowed him to trust me. I wondered if he would be shocked if he ever knew that I was someone he had loved for many years, and I had loved him back.

I was glad that I had taped that event and I watched it over and over again during the months that followed. I studied Walter and his every move. This was not an empty shell of a man, this was Dad at his finest. This was his home and these were his friends. We were not moving him to some other facility. Of that, I was damned sure. The staff had asked for a copy of the tape, which they played in the community room for the residents the following week. They were delighted and excited in seeing themselves and the other staff dancing on TV, reminiscent of the Lawrence Welk show, no doubt. Foot tapping could be seen and smiles emerged once again as the music on the tape started to play. I had a feeling that this was one tape I was going to treasure for a long, long time.

# XXII

# Empty Shadow Boxes

Most of my old friends were now gone, Andrew, Louis, Arthur, Stella and Eleanor. Their rooms were vacant, shadow boxes empty. My new friends and new experiences were waiting for me right down the road. The cycle of life waits for no one. Dr. Owen was the first to arrive. To me, he was a kindly looking old gent, always sporting a cap. He reminded me of a starched English gentleman. For some reason, I always noticed his shoes. He had a variety of highly polished very expensive looking shoes. I suppose it was a strange thing to notice about someone, but there you have it.

His new home was just down the hall from Dad's. Dr. Owen was also a very sad and troubled looking man. He would acknowledge me as I spoke to him, usually with a polite nod of his head, but never with words. I never ever heard him speak. He could talk though, as David had heard him speak many times in one- or two-word sentences, but just never to me. I noticed that he seemed to be a loner, and preferred to walk and sit by himself, reluctant to interact with the staff and other residents.

I took a walk toward his room, wondering how his family had pieced together his life in his shadow box. I'll bet he had an interesting and very exciting story. Hmmmmm . . . . Dartmouth College, class of 1942, Cornell

University School of Medicine 1945. It looked like he enjoyed fly fishing too. Several of the faded photos captured his moments of triumph as he sported his catch. What else had happened in his life? I could find no other particular clues in his shadow box. Oh yes . . . he had a dog. I didn't see any family photos, no holiday photos. No vacation photos either, just Dr. Owen and his dog.

Another brilliant mind, another nice person who had spent his whole life dedicated to the healing of other people. He must have felt betrayed at learning his own fate. Ignorance was not bliss for this poor highly educated man who knew better than anyone what was to lie ahead of him. He never seemed to be eating at meal time when we would visit, and I secretly wondered if this was part of his plan. He might take a bite or two and just push his plate away. It was at meal time that he would appear to be angry or disgusted. I wondered if he knew what was happening to him now, or if he was stuck in a world of confusion. I wondered if he knew he was a doctor. I wondered why he never had any visitors. I was worried about Dr. Owen. The cruel irony of life spares no one I guess.

Charles was an interesting man. I arrived one day to find him eating at Dad's table. I gave him my cheery "hello" and I told him that my name was "Janet." I always say that to all of my new friends and then I wait. I never know what to expect. Charles was different. His eyes seemed to follow you until you acknowledged him. They were friendly eyes. One could just tell. His facial expression was anxious, almost like he was desperately seeking conversation. "My name is Charles," he said, with a dignified Southern accent. He made it clear that his name was not "Charlie" or "Chuck," his name was "Charles." Secretly I was thinking, *My name is Janet . . . . J-A-N-E-T. Please remember my name.* My new friend Charles was an architect. He liked classical music, fine arts and history. Only five minutes have passed since I first met Charles and I have already bonded with him.

I tried to especially notice new residents and learn their names. Simply calling them by name usually seemed to make them feel better. The new faces were often sad. It must be a very upsetting thing to suddenly find yourself plunked down in the middle of this place, nice as it was. I would study their shadow boxes to get a tiny clue of something we could talk about. I wondered if they liked that, or wished I would go away instead of bothering them. It was very important to me to be able to make a small connection with each new resident in Dad's house. In some strange roundabout way, I was feeling like any little random act of kindness would find its way back to Dad in one form or another.

Herbert was a puzzle to me. Actually, it took me a little while to figure out that he was actually a resident. I met him in the resident living room one day, chatting away and introducing himself. He was very knowledgeable of current events, the world situation, the cost of this and that. He followed the stock market and he doled out advice to anyone who would listen. He was a very tall, thin man. He was well spoken and a fast talker. I found him to be especially interesting.

He looked sharp, sporting his pressed lightweight jacket and hat. He seemed to be waiting for someone, checking his watch several times as we spoke. At first I thought he must be just visiting a less fortunate friend or family member. It wasn't until we were leaving and making our way through the security doors that I noticed his picture hanging there with a message which read "Do not let this man out." I thought that surely there must be some kind of mistake. He seemed so active and with it mentally. Yes, he was interesting, very interesting and he was funny. He asked me my name.

I recalled how extremely irritating it was when Dad's friends would tell us how "great" Dad was. They were not looking at the big picture. This had to be the same kind of illusion. As time went on, we began to see the many sides of Herb. He had owned a successful manufacturing company and was a shrewd business man. He was very intelligent. He liked me and I could tell. He always came over to me to say hello. He always wanted to show me his garden. The facility allowed him a small garden patch and he was growing lovely fresh vegetables.

Whenever I would see Herb, his face would light up and he would immediately come toward us for a little visit. I would give him a hug and say "What's my name? . . . . What's my name?" He would always respond "Irene." "Herb . . . . what's my name?" He would smile and wink. "Janet," he would say. He never forgot . . . . never. There was something heartwarming about that, that he remembered my name. No one in this place ever remembered my name.

Herb spent most of his time studying the security doors. He figured out that a visitor would type in the security code on the key pad, and a clicking sound could be heard before they passed through the door. The door would actually remain unlocked for a few seconds before you could hear the loud click of the lock engaging again. As long as he was right on their heels, he calculated that he could make it through. Apparently, he was always making a break for it and could be found making his way down the road. He didn't actually have to make a break for it as I observed, he would simply blend in with the visitors. Most of the time they would hold the door for him.

He simply pretended he knew what he was doing. I found this to be very interesting and amusing in a small way. He was smart. It wasn't until a few months later before I understood the severity of his condition. There was a big argument going on in his room. He found one of the aides in there, collecting his laundry and all hell began to break loose. He flew into an extremely agitated and violent state. The loud angry voices were frightening to everyone. Nurses came running, his fists were flying and he ended up on the floor. He may have been a thin man, but he was a strong man and it took several of them to . . . . I could only assume, medicate him.

I was pretty sure he was not going to last long here, for the safety of the other residents. I was sure they were going to give him the boot. Where would he go? What would become of him? He was a nice man too. This was not his fault. He reacted that way because someone was taking his clothes. I was upset. I was upset for Herb, and I was upset for his poor family. They were about to get the "This behavior is unacceptable!" phone call. I wish I knew who they were. I wanted to talk to them. I would tell them it was okay. I wanted to tell them he was only protecting his stuff. Maybe Herb has already forgotten what happened. He probably forgot moments after it happened. The poor family has not forgotten, that much I am sure of.

A week later . . . I was surprised and relieved to see him, but from the time of that incident on, his personality seemed to have changed dramatically. Maybe it was new medication. Of course it was the medication. He walked around in a strangely calm, subdued state, but his spirit, his smile and even his personality appeared to be gone. He ate his meals without a word. He didn't really speak to anyone. His carefully groomed garden was now neglected. The plants drooped from lack of water. The tomatoes were rotting on the vines. I don't think he was trying to leave the facility anymore either. No more elaborate escape plans. His picture was no longer posted by each exit door. Everything was under control, behavior was modified. Isn't that just great? He never called me by name again.

# XXIII

## Shamrocks

I arrived one day to find two new kids on the block. They were a couple, and what a couple! I just loved this couple. Patrick and Katie were so perfectly Irish, they were almost a stereotype cliché. Patrick was a happy-go-lucky character. His bright blue eyes shone through his oversized thick glasses. He had the kind of face that was so cute, you just wanted to reach out and pinch his cheeks. He was bee-bopping down the corridor sporting his "Fighting Irish" sweatshirt. "Patrick, I just love your Fighting Irish shirt!" I said. He drew up his fists like a boxer, mimicking the cartooned fighter on his shirt.

He smiled a great big smile and chuckled. He knew perfectly well just how funny he was. His wife, Katie, was a perfect match for him. She adored him but could always hold her own, as she had been his sparring partner for over sixty years. He could still make her laugh. I really loved that. Katie was very petite and ladylike. Her hair was perfectly combed and she wore a light wool pink sweater set with pearl buttons. She traveled everywhere with her matching purse.

Somebody really loved their parents. I could tell by their lovely shadow boxes.

Katie often talked about their pride and joy, their only son Mike. Mike must have put together those beautiful tributes to his Mom and Dad. Maybe it was Mike's wife or a grandchild. Whoever it was, they really cared. I'm not sure what Patrick did later in life, but as a young man, he was the most handsome Army Officer I ever saw. His photo showed a U.S. Army Corps Pilot, later serving in the Reserves with the 905th Group. He was most proud of that.

Best of all, he was an Irishman to boot! Katie's photo was most glamorous and she was just beautiful. I told her all the time, "Katie, you had to be a movie star. You were beautiful then and you are beautiful now."

"Oh . . . go away with yourself," she would say, smiling and beaming with embarrassment. It was true, what a beautiful woman. What an awful thing to have both parents afflicted with Alzheimer's, but you know . . . I was so very glad that these two were in it together.

Patrick became Dad's buddy. I think it had to do with the fact that Dad would share his chocolates with him. Katie watched out for Dad, getting him to activities and whatnot. Patrick's condition was further advanced than Katie's, and she had her hands full keeping track of Patrick and now Dad too. She was not only beautiful, she was very motherly and sweet. The three of them could usually be found together. They ate all of their meals together too. Katie would insist that Patrick and Dad eat all of their peas. She would not allow the aide to deliver dessert until all plates were clean. The two men would make faces but in the end, they always obeyed her.

Patrick was funny. Dad would begin to get excited and would start to tell a story. He could never quite get it out. He would start over and over again and the thought pattern would drift off. Apparently it was a funny story as Dad would begin to laugh. Patrick would give Dad a most puzzled look, his face all scrunched up, as if to say "What the hell are you talking about, you daft bugger?" Patrick would whistle out

131

loud and make that "cuckoo" gesture with his finger rotating beside his head. He thought nothing of doing this right in front of Walter. Patrick was equally daft, and I say that with love. The best part was that the two of them could go on for hours entertaining each other. It wasn't important that none of us had any idea what either one of them was talking about.

Katie would just shake her head and roll her eyes. She would tell them both to shut up when she had enough, and they did. She was great. I recall we were having dinner with the three of them one night. David and I were talking over world events, news topics, politics and other riveting conversation to stimulate the three of them. I recall talking for a good long time, blessing them all with my vast knowledge and my unending opinions of world events, sports, weather and anything else I could think of.

When I was done, I noticed Patrick was staring at my hands. "What do you think, Patrick?" I asked.

After much thought he responded, "Looks nice."

"What looks nice, Patrick?" I asked.

"Pink" was his answer. He was looking at my pink nail polish. I could only laugh at my own foolishness. I thought I learned that lesson, to "be quiet and listen" a year and a half ago. Patrick reminded me of that. Simple . . . life is simple, be quiet and listen.

Patrick was easily amused. Someone once told me that I was easily amused, so perhaps that's why I liked him. I would see him in the hall, give him a giant wave and shout "Erin Go Braugh!" That was all it took to make his day. He would laugh for an hour. One day I happened to mention to Patrick that my cat was named "Patrick" too. I told him that it was obvious that my cat was both Irish and Catholic and he needed a good old Irish name for himself. Patrick thought that this was extremely amusing and he giggled for a good long time. He loved a little joke of any kind. He was always telling me that his room was filled with women. I would pretend that I was cross with him, shake my finger and sternly tell him that I was going to tell Katie. His eyes would open big and he would laugh some more.

Katie, hearing this for the umpteenth time, would take me by the hand and guide me down the hall to show me her room. Her expression told me she needed to help us both escape from daft men. Her walls were filled with photos, and her room was decorated very cheerfully, pink ruffles and most tidy. She would tell me more about her sweet son, her greatest gift in life. She was so proud of him. I asked her what he did for a living, but she seemed a little confused and could not remember. There were pictures of him all over her wall. The photographs seemed a little faded. I sure hope I get to meet him someday. If he was anything like his parents, he had to be a wonderful man.

Most of the new residents become annoyed as other residents would wander in and out of their rooms, touching and taking their belongings. Dad often talked about this, but I don't think he really notices it anymore. Katie was very irritated by other people wandering into her room at all hours of the night and day. She was troubled that there were no locks. She took me into her confidence and showed me her "booby trap." She closed her door and showed me this small set of wind chimes carefully tied to her door knob with yarn. This was her first line of defense, but there was more. There was "The Back-Up Plan." She showed me how she would carefully place a book on the floor, leaning it at an angle and just barely touching the door in exactly the right spot. If someone tried to open the door, the book would fall, the chimes would ring, and Katie could catch them red-handed.

I was pretty impressed with the whole thing, especially the part about the "Back-Up Plan." "Katie," I said, "let's give it a try." She got very excited over the whole testing of her plan thing. First she looked up and down the hall. It was important that no one knew what we were up to. I went outside her room and she closed the door. I could hear shuffling and jingling sounds going on in there. A minute or so later, I heard a little voice say "Okay . . . come on in!" I slowly and carefully turned the knob and gave the door a little push. Chimes began to ring, "thud," there went the book. There sat Katie on the edge of her bed with a big smile. She was shaking her finger at me and she sang with glee, "I caught you!!!"

Like Herb, Katie and Patrick would sit for hours studying the exit door. I came in one day and Katie patted the chair seat next to her, inviting me to sit down. She and Patrick almost had the whole thing worked out but she needed my help. Patrick began by telling me that all of the people who leave here are reaching into the bush by the door and are pulling something out. This, he deducted, is what makes the door open. Katie corrected him, telling him that there was a secret combination thing with numbers on it behind the bush, and you needed to press the right numbers . . . then the door would open.

She was pretty accurate about that, except for what was on the other side of the door. She told me of this whole elaborate floor plan with various floors, stairs and elevators, twists and turns which needed to be maneuvered through before you could actually escape to the parking lot. In reality, it was a rather simple floor plan all on one level, but still, she was thinking. "Honey . . . " she said to me, "I was thinking that you could tell me which numbers I need to push to get that door to open."

"Oh Katie . . . " I said, "I don't know what the numbers are either." I lied.

She looked at me sadly for a minute or two and then leaned over and whispered in my ear. "Don't you worry, Honey . . . when I find out what they are, I'm going to tell you." She patted my hand and gave me a wink. What a sweet woman.

Once in a while David would visit Dad without me, sometimes during the day while I was at work. Katie didn't like that one bit. She would always ask where I was. She would tell David to make sure that I came with him the next time. She sternly reminded him how important it was that we visited more often too. When I came to visit, I was greeted by her warm and wonderful smile. "I was just thinking that you were going to come for a visit with me! Let's sit down for a minute and chat. Let me show you my room and all of my pictures."

"That sounds great, Katie," I would respond. I would follow her down the hall to her room, pausing for a moment at her shadow box. I would always point to her lovely picture. "Who is that beautiful movie star?" I waited for her response, that slightly embarrassed expression and her genuine smile. "Oh . . . go away with you!" she would giggle.

Patrick was in the mood for ice cream, and so naturally, Dad was too. Patrick was getting his coat on because Dad told him I would take them out for some. They didn't understand that I couldn't simply just drive off with the residents. Two sad, little boy faces were looking back at me. I went down the hall to ask the nurse if Patrick and Katie were allowed to have ice cream sundaes. She smiled and answered "Yes!" Back down the hall I went to find sad-faced Patrick. "Patrick . . . if you go put on my favorite 'Fighting Irish' sweatshirt, I'll go out and get you an ice cream sundae." His face lit up, he turned and trotted down the hall to his room. I drove off to Friendly's for three hot fudge sundaes to go.

# XXIV

## Where America Loves to Shop

Alright, where is my list? Why is it, I can never find my damned list? I searched my purse. I searched my coat pockets. Ironic isn't it? I'm pretty sure that Gingko was on the top of that list, at least I think it was, I don't really remember. Ah . . . another relaxing trip to Wal-Mart. David remembered that cleaning supplies were on that list and toothpaste- . . . yah . . . toothpaste, but that was it. Twenty items on the missing list and that was the best we could do. I took a deep breath. Alright, let's just go in. Maybe I'll get a brainstorm once we get in there. I asked David to take charge of the cart. He was going one way, and me the other. By now we were getting excited. We were up to six items that we remembered. That's not too bad. Great, now we are lowering our own bar of acceptance.

While David was filling up the cart with some sweatshirts he needed for work, I was busy running up and down the aisles in search of shampoo and toothpaste. I like to load up on this stuff so I don't have to return back to this place where all of America loves to shop too often. With my arms loaded, each item carefully stacked and balanced, I made my way here, there and everywhere in search of David and the cart. David was proudly showing me some new shoe laces which he was going to buy. I tossed my armloads of stuff in to the cart and pretended to be excited for him. He was headed off with the cart to look at leather work boots for himself, also new underwear and Velcro laced sneakers for Dad. I was off to stock up on the cleaning supplies and antacid pills . . . see you in a few minutes.

I again searched for David and the cart, arms again loaded and this time aching. Hmmm . . . Not in the boot section, not in the underwear section. David remembered that we needed cat food and was busy tossing in an undetermined number of cans. "Do you think twenty-four cans are enough?" Who cares, let's go. David was going to the automotive section and then off to pick up some film. I forgot the Tylenol . . . gotta go back for the big bottle. Thinking that we pretty much had covered the items on the missing list, I took a deep breath and took my time as I gazed at all of the pain relievers, neatly arranged . . . so many choices. I was searching for zinc cream for Dad's arms, and special shower wash for him, when I was startled by the sight of David, clutching a roll of film in his hand. "Are we almost ready to get out of here?" he asked cheerfully.

I looked in front of him . . . nothing. I looked behind him . . . nothing. I looked beside him . . . nothing. "David . . . what did you do with the cart?"

He looked puzzled. "Me? . . . I thought you had the cart."

Bloody hell. The word Alzheimer's popped into my head. Okay, take me to the pillow aisle so I can smother myself. Dear God, I am pretty sure I can not do this Alzheimer's thing again. I questioned David on where he had been, but he wasn't sure. We tried retracing his steps. That didn't work either. We searched for a good twenty minutes or so before I came across our cart, sitting there all alone in the candy aisle. That figures, I should have checked there first. All of our stuff was piled high in the cart. It was a good thing I decided not to throw my purse in there with David in charge. We checked out and I walked silently back to the car as David pushed the cart.

I was secretly watching him out of the corner of my eye. I didn't want him to get lost on the way to the car with all of our stuff. Good thing I bought the big bottle of Tylenol. Where are my keys? God . . . get me out of this place. I checked my purse and began shoving my hands into my pockets. What's this in the back pocket of my jeans? It was my list. What was it doing in there? I never shove things in my back pocket. I studied it for a moment. Crap . . . I forgot the freaking Gingko. I am thinking that God has an interesting sense of humor.

# XXV
## Summer Wedding Bells

Raymond called us with the great news. He was getting married. It was the second marriage for the both of them so they were keeping it simple. It was to be a small wedding next month with immediate family and a few close friends. It was really nice to have the phone ring, followed by good news. It seems like so long ago since that happened. Ray was wondering if we should bring Dad. We all felt as though Dad wouldn't realize what was going on, but still, you should have your father there on your wedding day. I thought it would be nice for them to have Dad in all of the family wedding photos too.

We told Ray that we would pick up Dad and look after him during the wedding and reception, and we would bring him back to his home when Dad decided it was time to go. I started to wonder if our half-hearted attempts were self serving, merely to pick up a few extra brownie points with God. Maybe we were actually getting demerits for torturing Dad by keeping up appearances, dragging him off to each of these family gatherings when we knew perfectly well, that he didn't want to be away from his surroundings.

We arrived early to pick up Dad. We got him dressed in a clean and pressed shirt with elastic waistband pants. We packed a bag with extra clothes and "Daddy Diapers" just in case. We had brought a wedding card for him to sign, and David sat down with him to see what we could do about getting him to sign "Love, Dad" on the card. David would quietly repeat each letter of the brief message several times as Dad began to write.

Dad placed the pen on the card and began to draw what was to be a large clockwise drawn letter "O." It was interesting to me, and I wondered if Walter's brain was actually seeing the letters that he was repeating. Starting at the top, he would repeat each letter that David was telling him, but just continue around with the pen until the large and shaky "O" was complete. "There," he announced with satisfaction. We placed the card in the envelope and made our way to church.

We coached Dad on the details of the who's, what's, where's and when's of the nuptial adventure, but to no avail; he really wasn't understanding. He seemed uneasy as we buckled him into the seat. He frequently announced that we had been driving for a long time. It was about a half hour drive, but I had to agree with him; it seemed like forever. We finally arrived. He seemed uneasy at first being around loud happy strangers, but eventually became more comfortable.

The ceremony began. It was being held in this beautiful little country church. The bride and groom recited their vows. They were personal and very heartfelt vows and there was not a dry eye in the place. The ceremony was lovely. About halfway through, Walter began looking around, somewhat distracted. He started to get up but he sat back down. Then he began to fiddle with his program and was flipping through the hymnal.

I reached out and I grabbed his hand firmly. *I am not leaving and neither are you,* I thought. I almost said the words sternly out loud but luckily I stopped myself. *Great,* I thought. *Not only am I being mean to a poor old man with Alzheimer's who*

140

*didn't really want to be here in the first place, but also I am being mean to him in church.* That's got to be bad. I should have been paying attention to the ceremony but instead my mind digressed to "The Care Givers Burnout List" which I had read years ago.

It was item number six on the list which bothered me. Out of ten items listed, the only item I couldn't answer "Yes" to was item number six. It read, "(6) Do you have outbursts of anger at you loved one with Alzheimer's when he or she behaves erratically or becomes difficult?" Before today, I could always answer "No." It looks like I completed all of the items on the burnout list. There was that tight pain again, burning its way up the back of my neck. We sat quietly, hand in hand until the ceremony was over. I apologized to God . . . again.

We all got Dad into as many photographs as we could and headed back to Ray's house for a small reception. Dad joined right in with the festivities, he smiled and laughed in all the right places. He tried to join in on conversations, but you could see that the thought patterns became interrupted. He would begin to tell a story, but he would just fade away. People would just smile and say, "Oh, that's nice, Walter." Then they would make a quick getaway to avoid any embarrassing moments perhaps. He asked a few times, where he was, why he was there, and when was he going back. Dad's old furry and faithful friend "Jake" made a guest appearance, as this had become his new home when Walter was moved to the facility a few years before. Dad didn't seem to acknowledge him.

We decided to start back home. Too bad, I really wanted a bite of cake. They hadn't cut it yet but Dad wanted to leave. Quietly, we made our exit and started the drive back to Dad's home. Our thoughts were interrupted as Dad excitedly pointed to the sunset. It was beautiful. Dad talked about it over and over again and he followed it with keen excitement all the way home. Dad had taken pictures of beautiful sunsets his whole life. His albums were full of them. Yet, it was as if he were seeing a sunset for the very first time. Maybe it was the very first time for him. The very first time he was seeing it from the perspective of his new world.

It took Dad to remind us of the simple beauties in life. We pulled up to the front door of his facility. It was a welcoming sight for us, although Dad seemed surprised that this was his home, and we needed to explain that it was. He thought it was quite large and impressive. We punched in the security code and went through the doors. We signed him back in and got him ready for bed. The other residents were already asleep. I wondered if Dad had enjoyed his outing. I had the idea that it was already forgotten. We were still not ready to accept his world. We still insisted on forcing him into our world. Each time with each attempt, we become more disappointed and more frustrated. Every time, we secretly planned to try again.

# XXVI

## Happy Birthday Dear Dad . . .
## Happy Birthday to Youuuuu . . .

Dad is turning seventy-eight . . . what do we do. Our family loves a good party and we always enjoyed turning almost any occasion into an event. My first thought was to plan a giant to-do at our home. We could invite everyone we know. Any excuse to get him out of that home and bring him here. I am constantly striving to recreate memories of the old days, the happy days of large gatherings, plenty of food and laughter and lots of love. I decided that these re-creations lately were more for our benefit than for Dad's. We are very slow learners indeed. Luckily, Dad is patient with us. He is able to persevere calmly while we continue to learn.

A few weeks ago we had decided to take Dad out for ice cream. For as many years as I can remember, he always enjoyed our almost nightly rides in the summer down the back county roads as the black Buick made its way to a little farm which made the world's best homemade "creamers" as Dad would say. Wanting to keep those memories alive, one particular hot summer night we arrived at Dad's home with a plan. After repetitive coaxing, he finally agreed to use the bathroom.

We dressed Walter in a nice clean shirt and combed his hair. He looked nice. This was going to be great!!! We signed him out, maneuvered through the maze of security doors and slowly made our way to the parking lot, trying to build up his enthusiasm with stories of our "creamer adventures" from long ago. Although he was initially agreeable, I could feel that this little outing was more about us . . . again.

We carefully buckled him in and began to drive the drive we took so many times before. Dad repeatedly questioned where we were going and was apprehensive about leaving his environment, confused and worried about returning. It was only a fifteen minute drive, a drive which was raising everyone's blood pressure. Dad continued to tell us that this was a "very long drive."

The beautiful country road, the houses and farms had somehow lost their appeal for me. The ice cream tasted different that day, not the way I remembered it at all, and it was a relief to return to the welcoming doors of his home. Not the perfect plan and perhaps I was just trying to lessen the little guilt pains I have been having by my infrequent visits lately.

His reluctance to leave his surroundings and his constant worry about returning to his home, in addition to our now worrying about his "Daddy Diapers," extra clothes we needed on hand for him in case of accidents, not to mention the fact that I was now rehearsing interesting dialog in advance as a way to convince him that he would have a great time every time we took him out, was becoming a chore. Can I believe I was now saying "chore," what kind of a person was I anyway? I remember a year or two earlier when I was so proud of myself for my ability to listen to him and hear what he was communicating, even if it was in his own special way.

He hasn't known me for about nine or ten months now. I am still a nice lady . . . the lady who brings him chocolates . . . that he remembers, and I am good with that. He hasn't really seemed to acknowledge David as his son, or call him by name for about two months or so, although after several reminders with each visit he seems to come around a bit. I'm sure he still feels that he is connected to David in some way, but one can see that he just isn't quite sure how. He is sweet though, and I smile as you can see he is very careful about not hurting anyone's feelings. He still picks up on little cues to keep the conversations flowing.

His life is very simple now. A structured simple routine that he is comfortable with, in a friendly, safe and clean environment. David called the home several days before his birthday and asked if it might be possible to bring a little party to him, instead of taking him away. The staff was more than receptive and offered us the choice of two indoor areas of the facility for our party. We chose the one which resembled an outdoor French bistro café, street lamps, bistro tables and wall fountains included.

We contacted only those most close to Walter, fourteen in all and asked if they would join us. They all asked what would be appropriate to bring as a gift. As Dad had all he really needed, we suggested that if they wanted to bring something for him, to only bring something simple, something very small and simple. That morning we packed up our supplies, our plates and flatware, napkins and cleaning stuff and ordered some pizza which we picked up on the way. Raymond and his family were bringing the cake, chips and soda. Joan was bringing the ice cream. Smiles in place . . . off we go.

We arrived a little early to set up the bistro area and David went to fetch Dad and gussy him up a bit for his visitors. Walter did not realize it was his birthday and looked a little vague as guests arrived, but it wasn't long before his wit and charm kicked right in. He lit up with recognition as his two very special lifelong friends arrived. He knew their names. It was amazing. I watched as he smiled and laughed as his close circle of family and friends rallied around him.

I was my usual somewhat intrusive self, snapping pictures wherever possible, still trying to capture each moment. The candles on the cake were lit and singing rang down the hallways. Walter joined right in singing the "happy birthday" chorus, as he still wasn't quite sure whose birthday it was. Walter's brother leaned forward to help him blow out his candles.

Today was different. There was something so sweet about the way he seemed at ease in his own environment. This was his home, this was now, and we were not trying to recreate festivities of the past. His close friends and family were celebrating with him, for him in his own world. His own new friends, other residents wandered in when they heard the singing, and were offered cake and ice cream to celebrate with Walter, waiting long enough, of course for me to run down the hall and check with the powers-that-be to make sure their diets allowed this.

During the celebration, Walter's youngest son Jackie, called from Florida to wish him a happy birthday. He seemed confused and actually put the phone down and wandered away while they were still speaking to him. David had to run over and direct him to pick up the phone and continue listening. I stood on the sidelines and watched as Walter's gifts were piled in front of him.

Each card and gift were those of a most precious kind. David helped Walter open each card, and slowly read every sentiment out loud to his Dad. Walter struggled a bit with opening his packages. The simplicity of the most perfect gifts touched me. Small handpicked boxes of his very favorite chocolates, homemade fancy cookies . . . just exactly what he loved, photos of happy memories his friends had shared with Walter years ago, and a beautiful rose which his brother had grown for him in his garden.

Dad still didn't know me that day, but he did say I looked a little familiar. I told him that was because I was a famous movie star and I had heard that it was his birthday. I told him I flew in from Hollywood just to give him a birthday kiss. He smiled that wonderful smile and his eyes twinkled. ''Happy Birthday, Dad . . . I love you,'' I whispered softly. I smiled and looked at his face. I was still learning things from that wonderful man. Everything that was most important to him was happening right now and could be found right there in that little bistro. It was as simple as that.

# XXVII

# Accelerating Downhill
# on the Road of Life . . .
# and the Brakes Aren't Working

It's been over three years now since Mom died. I found it almost an effort to visit Walter. I understood the routine. It was always the same. Walter would show another tiny sign of progression toward the advanced phase and I would analyze it for a week, lower the bar of acceptance again and wait for the next sign. We would now silently make the drive to Dad's facility. We would exchange pleasantries with the staff at the front desk and sign in on the guest register. We would squirt a small dab of hand disinfectant in our palms as requested by the facility and with smiles in place we would proceed through the security doors.

We would find Walter. We would make our usual stroll up and down the hallway. We would chit-chat about the weather. We would talk about how he is feeling these days. Dad would tell us that they have been moving his room again. We would show him his room, and he would tell us that they must have moved it back. Sometimes I would bring in photos to show Dad what we had been up to lately.

We would give him a detailed account of what had been going on in the lives of all the family members. Dad would appear interested, but we can see he has no idea who we are talking about. We would pause for a moment to look in his shadow box. Dad didn't know any of the faces in his shadow box anymore. He didn't recognize his mother or his father. The pictures of his Navy ship were a mystery and I felt sad as I could see the shadows of his life fading away one by one.

Walter didn't seem to know David anymore, or at least he was not calling him by name. Sometimes he would give David a look of recognition, and sometimes not. David had given him a sweatshirt with our family name on it and Dad had said it was very nice. He didn't make the connection with himself and the family name. He looked at the shirt for a while, and then told us he hoped he didn't have to give it back. He thought for a little while longer with a worried expression and said that he hoped he didn't owe anyone money for it. David repeatedly told him that it was his shirt and he didn't owe anyone any money. A few minutes would pass and he would express his concerns again.

I heard the old familiar sound of a whizzing walker. Tilly raced by, her face was all black and blue. I was shocked as I looked at her face. It wasn't what I would describe as slight bruising or discoloration. Something very bad had happened to her and the blue-black color was deep and dark. The bruises covered her entire face. I felt a rush of fear and a pain in my stomach as I flashed back to that terrible February, and the horrible incident of Dad slapping some nice little old lady. Maybe Tilly had fallen. I called out her name, twice . . . she didn't answer, she just kept rolling. He eyes fixed straight ahead of her.

We went to Dad's room. The smell of urine was no longer shocking to me. It was just like any other day. Dad's barricade in front of his radiator had been moved again. There was a puddle on the floor. The sign which read "TOI-LET" on his bathroom door fell down again and I didn't bother to tape it back up. Page forty-two of the new book I am reading says to "praise the person when he or she uses

the bathroom successfully." It all sounded pretty condescending to me.

Walter was not a child. He can not correct this behavior
at will and he would never want to know that this was his
new behavior, although the book says differently. It says that
many people with Alzheimer's remain acutely aware of their
deficiencies, and we should not embarrass them by showing
distaste. I do not believe it. He is not aware of his deficiencies. I certainly would never do anything to embarrass Walter
under any circumstances, but I am telling you . . . he is not
aware of his deficiencies.

We had complained to the staff that Dad's shaver was
missing again, and I had an uncontrollable urge to search
each of the resident's rooms until I could get my hands on
the culprit who stole it. The staff searched every room. The
missing shaver was eventually found in the pocket of Dad's
own winter coat. It was late summer. What was it doing in
the pocket of his winter coat which was carefully stowed away
in the back of his closet? I don't know. Anyway, why was it
that his shaver always stopped working when it needed to be
cleaned? Dad would walk around unshaven for days, until
we arrived to clean his shaver. Who was cleaning the shavers
of the poor old souls without family members who keep their
watchful eyes opened?

Why were some of his framed photographs missing and
what about his belt? He had been walking around the place
with his pants falling down for weeks now. Where the hell
was the belt? Again we made a big stink and had the staff
scurrying around in search of his belt. I personally searched
every inch of his room and it was not there. A few days later,
I was cleaning out my car and my jaw dropped as I opened
a crumpled paper bag in my trunk. It was the bag of extra
clothes we had brought to Ray's wedding a month or so ago.
There was his belt. The right thing to do would have been

to immediately drive over to Dad's place and apologize to the staff. I didn't.

A few weeks had gone by since I last went to visit Walter. It was long past the time to make the journey again. I wondered if it really mattered to Dad or anyone else that I was going. Silently, I drove there, stopping once for a small box of chocolates. I saw some new people at the facility. New, sad and lonely faces. They were just starting this phase of their journey. I didn't know their names. I wasn't sure I wanted to know their names and I didn't even want to see their shadow boxes. I quietly sneaked passed Patrick's and Katie's rooms. I just didn't feel like being cheerful today. Great . . . now I'm bringing down the poor, old, already sad people. I remember a time when I used to feel so great when I was able to make them smile.

The last time I was there, I saw Katie. Katie didn't know me that day. It was the first time since I had met her that she didn't remember me. You would think that I would be used to that kind of thing by now, but I'm not. Katie said that I looked familiar, and she wanted to know just who I was. "My name is Janet," I said softly with my eyes fixed to the floor. She had that inquisitive look on her face like I was meeting her for the first time. If one more person I care about tells me, "You look familiar," I am going to scream.

Since then, I had been doing some more reading to prepare ourselves for our next hurdle in life . . . The Advanced Phase. The article said "Inability to use language, becoming easily disoriented, incontinence, walking with a shuffle, showing minimal emotional response, immobility and pain, weight loss, inability to swallow, agitation, paranoia, more mood changes, difficulty sleeping." Dad can no longer tie his shoes. His gait is now much slower, more like a very slow shuffle. His doctor found skin cancer on back of his neck which required surgery.

He now has a terrible rash on both arms and on parts of his legs. He is supposed to have special zinc medication applied several times a day. I wonder if that is happening. The irritation was made worse by his constant scratching. I had asked his doctor to run a culture on his open wounds, as I was convinced that the hand washing in the toilet thing had given him some awful disease. He was instead diagnosed with severe dermatitis. I guess that was supposed to be good news. He also now suffers from swollen legs due to some kind of valve malfunction in his veins and the fluid is beginning to pool.

He was fitted for special hose to improve circulation. We arrived to find the staff has again put the special hose on the wrong legs. Jesus . . . we labeled them "Left" and "Right" for a reason. Each leg has its own measurements and each hose has a different prescription. The tongues of his sneakers are not pulled up correctly again either. They are jammed way down inside the toe of the shoe. That's got to hurt. Did they just shove his feet in the shoes that way and leave them, or what? I can not believe they didn't notice. Is it really so difficult to dress him with a little care? Maybe Dad had dressed himself that morning, but they could have checked. I know they have their hands full but for God's sake, they have the doctor's written orders on file.

The book says that it is important to build positive relationships with the staff, keeping in mind that there are days with unforeseen circumstances, such as short staffing. The book says to try to not take it out on those who are there. The book says to give praise too, don't forget to let the staff know when you are pleased, when things are going right. Am I supposed to say "Congratulations and good job for getting his socks and shoes on the right feet today?" "Thanks a million for finally applying this medication to his arms and legs as instructed by the doctor." My keen sense of observation tells me that no one really cares. "Dad . . . let's straighten out your shoes and socks . . . Okay?"

I have seen no particular noticeable improvement in the cognitive memory which they spoke of from the new drug which was prescribed for Dad, but the staff says it's working great. Maybe it is great. Maybe it's just me, but I am not seeing anything. I'm not a professional, I guess. I don't know what I expected to see. I went to the seminars, I know how it goes. We are not hearing anything more about the sedative which was prescribed for him to lessen agitation and we don't ask.

We have not received any more "This behavior is unacccptable" phone calls of late so I guess I can only assume the sedative is doing its job. I guess everything here is under control. I kiss Dad goodbye, and he looks startled. For one very brief fleeting second, I had a feeling that Dad might lash out at me. I was actually afraid, just for that one brief second. I was afraid of this kind and gentle man. Was it that he was afraid of me? What was happening? Was it real or imagined?

Another family gathering night was arranged by the staff. The invitation arrived. We can always count on festive music and wonderful food anyway. I must say that this facility does one heck of a job when it comes to planning and orchestrating family events. One of the nurses was excited to show us Dad's art work. The residents had been painting, and their work was on display. Dad had been a pretty good painter during his lifetime. He especially loved to paint sunsets and pictures of the sand dunes and ocean seascape memories of Cape Cod. He even had one of his oil originals hanging in his room at the facility which he had painted maybe forty years ago. We made our way to the community room in search of Dad's creations. I was very excited and curious to see what Dad had done.

There were three paintings which Dad had done. Each one with a brilliant blue background, each one with a small blotch of brown paint at the bottom right hand corner. The background color and images appeared only on the right hand side of each painting. The left half of the canvas was completely blank. It was as if someone had drawn an imaginary line right down the middle of the canvas. I looked at all three. Each was identical. What did that mean? What was happening to the right side of his brain to make the left side of his painting completely vacant? I'll bet there are volumes of documentation which would tell me about the ganglion fibers in one's brain which would account for this interesting phenomenon.

My thoughts returned once again to the Reagan family. Twenty years of courage and commitment. People talk about it but I wondered if they really understood what that family was going through. When people talk about them with admiration, were they really feeling it and did they have a true understanding or was it empty sentiment? I'm thinking it was not empty sentiment. It was an outpouring of heartfelt, sincere sentiment perhaps without full understanding. Maybe it was a full understanding which I was not seeing.

Do people realize that the family members who lived every day of their lives with a loved one affected by this disease were heroes? I often see other resident's family members. We smile politely at each other as we pass in the hallway. It's as if we belong to some secret society of our own. Sometimes they seem surprised when I call their father or mother by name. Were they feeling the same thing that I was feeling every time they visited, or were they much stronger and more accepting than me? It didn't matter anyway I guess, I am who I am.

The topic of money is rearing its ugly head again. Dad's commercial property has still not been sold. We have a realtor helping us with it but this saga still continues after several years. Taxes still need to be paid, and maintenance still needs to be done. We have started inquiring on the procedure to get Dad into a local nursing home sometime down the road. We were advised to look at his finances carefully. The cost of a nursing home is almost double the cost of where he is now.

The nursing homes will accept Title 19, but is was strongly suggested that we plan to have at least a year or two worth of payments in the bank. It was inferred that he would move up on the waiting list faster if he were a paying customer. What happens to all of those poor people who worked so hard their whole life, only to find that their money was gone that first year? What if they have no money at all? Was there just one aspect of this whole process which I might understand, without an endless flood of more questions to follow?

Some people have told me that their parent was accepted immediately into a nursing facility, without assets and already qualified under Title 19. Others have stated, that depending on the facility itself, the rules could be quite different. It was during that conversation that it was communicated, shall we say, that one could move up the waiting list much quicker if he or she were a paying customer. Apparently, after being an established paying patient at a nursing home for a couple of years, the nursing home would be obliged to accept Title 19 once the funds ran out. Other people have told us that sometimes you need to fight with them and demand that they keep your loved one once the money runs out. That figures. More turmoil to come with the next phase. More corporate baloney. I can't wait to get a peek at their brochures.

How were we supposed to plan for this anyway? Will he need to move next year, or five years from now? What happens if five years turns into ten? The commercial property is like a huge anchor around our necks. The sale would have meant that Dad would be taken care of for several more years at least. On paper, it looks like Dad has a lot of assets. In reality, there are problems with the property that are hindering the sale. Depending on how you look at it, it is either a valuable asset or a worthless liability. This does not fit at all on the tidy Financial Worksheet given to us.

My thoughts returned to Dad and that one cold winter afternoon several years ago. That was the day he told us he saw a man on TV with Alzheimer's and he said that if he were that man, he would pick the coldest day of the year to go for a walk, and he would just keep walking. We were so shocked and horrified at the message he was sending us. Was it possible that maybe he knew what was happening to him? Did he possess a wisdom far beyond our understanding and could it have been that he did not want to be a burden to his family? It would have been just like Dad to think of us first. I began to wonder what I would have done if I had been in his shoes.

Knowing what I now know and watching these poor souls and their downward progression have changed my views on a couple of things. I have some very strong beliefs, but they are very personal beliefs and I share them only with God. I have very strong opinions on what is right and what is wrong. These opinions change frequently, but I'm pretty sure God understands. There is no other way to say this except to say that I completely respect the feelings and decisions of anyone afflicted with a terminal condition. Living with the hopeless knowledge of one's own horrible ending has to be a terrible burden to bear.

I always have a thousand questions, but I always feel completely inadequate when it comes to finding the answers. I have a tendency to not let things go, ever. I can talk about my belief in the bigger picture, God's plan, the lessons in life I need to learn, all things happening for a reason, and things like that. Although I believe in all of these things, my mind is still constantly working overtime searching for the answers. Even in my sleep, I am still hashing it all out. I am even getting on my own nerves with my quest to have an organized approach to every detail in life. Imagine how I am affecting my poor family members who have to be exposed to me each day. I hope I am not damaging their tapestries. Maybe someday I will acquire the courage and the wisdom needed to be comfortable with simple acceptance. Today is not that day.

Today is a day that I have to remind myself that God, too, has a sense of humor. What else could it be? The day began like any other. I was deep in thought, pondering the meaning of life and whatnot as I stood peering in the mirror. I was in a hurry as I was getting ready for work. You know, for a woman approaching fifty, I didn't look half bad. No . . . I looked great! I recently got myself a nice new hair-cut, and my hair dresser took out all of the grey. I was really feeling better about myself.

I bought myself one of those at-home micro-dermabrasion exfoliator kits. The name itself sounded pretty impressive and the label on the box said I could scrub years off of my sorry, saggy, weathered and wrinkled face with constant use. I don't think those were the exact words the marketing department came up with to use on the box, but that was the gist of it. Nonetheless, it seemed to be working. It was fall again, and I had gone shopping. I found a beautiful light pumpkin colored sweater with tiny buttons. It was pretty, and it looked great with my black trousers. Hmmmm . . . black makes me look skinny. Yep . . . I looked great.

My mind was in its usual whirl, planning out my work-day. Gotta do this . . . gotta do that. I wonder what is going on with Walter and I must go and visit him after work. That recent whole bureaucratic nursing home conversation was weighing heavily on my mind. I still may have had years before I needed to worry about it, but for some reason I had chosen to worry about it now. I continued with mentally organizing my day as I quickly applied my makeup. I'm not really sure what happened next.

I must have had my open stick of mascara in my hand as I contemplated whether that sweater should be tucked in or left out. I decided to try it in. I stood in front of the mirror, and changed my mind, no, it looks better out. I started to pull it out when to my horror, the image looking back at me had black ink all over the bottom of my beautiful new sweater. "What the hell???" I pulled some more . . . black ink all over the place. I gave my sweater one last pull.

Out popped the opened mascara stick. It fell to the floor. Now there was a black trail on the tile as the stick made a few bounces before it finally came to a rest. "Bloody Hell!!!" I yelled as I realized that in my haste, I had apparently tucked the opened mascara stick into my pants along with the sweater. I looked back into the mirror. I was shocked. How could I be so incredibly stupid? How could I have done that? How could I have done something like that without knowing? Do I laugh or cry . . . laugh . . . cry . . . laugh . . . cry . . . which one? I wanted to choose cry, but time was running out and I had to get cleaned up and go. No time to cry right now. I made a mental note that I shall save that for later as I ponder what the hell was going on with my own tangled ganglion brain fibers.

I decided that if a professional were to perform a scan of my brain this very minute, they would have had to call out their colleagues in great droves. Instead of finding the usual grey matter and other assorted brain tissue, they would be amazed to see the image of a large void with one lone dimly lit light bulb. Perhaps they would see the frantic bug buzzing around the light, haphazardly and repeatedly bumping into the bulb as it continued its great mission of God knows what. It would be a medical amazement. They would scratch their heads, in search of a gene that controls the production of protein in the brain. It's known as stathmin or oncoprotein 18 and is associated with anxiety. I think my number 18 is broken.

Okay. So what's the big deal. Who hasn't done something scatterbrained once or twice a week? I seem extremely sensitized these days to any signs of daftness. I secretly wonder if I had been doing things like that for years and just never noticed. Perhaps I should just retire to Bedlam and call it a day. This is worrisome, however I'm sure my mind just has too many things whirling around in there at once. No big deal. I'll just carry on as usual. I will now put myself behind the wheel of a three thousand pound motor vehicle and hope to God that I have my own Guardian Angel as my back seat driver today. Crap . . . where did I put my keys?

# XXVIII

## Big Stakes Gambling

Today I shall have a greater understanding of all of those around me. Today I shall accept things as they come. Today I shall slow down and smell the roses. Today I shall go forth and visit Walter. I have a feeling that just maybe I will learn something new today. Dad was not in his room. I made my way down the hall to the dining area. There seemed to be a big card game going on down there. There was Walter, deep in thought, scratching his head and studying his hand. Walter and Anne used to set aside Friday night as card night in their home for many years. Friends and relatives would turn it into an event each week with lots of food and wine, lots of laughter.

This should be interesting. Walter was sitting at the table with Patrick and Herb. I was glad to see that Herb had joined in. I had been worried about him lately. There was a new fellow too. His name was William, or "Bill the Barber" as they called him. Apparently Bill had owned and operated a barber shop in town for nearly forty years. Bill reminded me a lot of my own father. He was funny and was very opinionated. Bill knew everyone and everything about everyone in town. I was glad that Bill found his way into this tight little circle of friends. They were playing poker for cookies. Walter, Herb and Bill had meager piles of only two maybe three cookies each. Patrick, on the other hand had a huge pile carefully stacked up in front of him.

I watched with interest as events began to unfold. This was a game that I was not familiar with. Each man took his turn drawing a card and then discarding. There did not appear to be either rhyme or reason to the cards in their hands. Every time it was Patrick's turn, he would draw a card, let out a laugh, and proudly lay down his hand for all to see. He would then quickly scoop up his opponents cookies and announce that he had won again. No one challenged him. They were in complete acceptance. Now, I am no card wiz, but one could clearly see that no two cards in his hand had anything in common. Nonetheless, his was apparently a winning hand. His other worthy opponents would let out a sigh, shake their heads and say "better luck next time" to each other.

Patrick was delighted with himself and clearly knew he was cheating. At least I think he knew he was cheating. Yes, I am sure my friend Patrick knew he was cheating. He asked me if I wanted to play. I smiled at him and told him that I was on to his shenanigans. He flashed me back a giant smile and gave me a wink. He knew that I would not spill the beans. At least I think he knew I wouldn't spill the beans. The game continued until all of the cookies were in Patrick's possession. Patrick claimed victory and the sad but worthy adversaries admitted defeat and went their separate ways. Dad made his way back down the hall, shaking his head, repeating that Patrick was really good, and that he was a tough one to beat . . . really good.

Walter stopped in the hall and took my hand. He thought for a moment before he spoke. "You know . . . You should never bet any more than you can afford to lose. Come to think of it, it's probably better if you don't gamble at all." The words came out as clear as a bell. "Dad," I said, "that is some really good advice. I am always going to remember that you told me that." He smiled and we continued hand in hand down the hall. On my way home that night, I stopped at the store. I needed to pick Dad up his own bag of "Chips Ahoy" chocolate chip cookies which he loved so much.

I arrived back home, still smiling as I remembered how Dad had lovingly given me that important advice. I looked in my mail box. Hmmmm. The usual mound of junk mail, all except for this exciting letter from Ed McMahon. Looks like I may have won a million dollars again . . . that is good news. Wait a minute, I got a letter from my Aunt Mary who lives out of state. She is a wonderful sweet woman who always sends me cards.

Let's see, nope, it's not my birthday. Our anniversary was months ago, and no holidays were on the horizon. I wonder what's going on. Aunt Mary's cards always cheer me up. I couldn't wait to tear open the envelope. It seems that it was their fiftieth wedding anniversary. Damn, I felt a pain of remorse as I had forgotten to send her a card. She told me that she had always wanted to visit the relatives in Ireland, and that her kids had given them a trip as an anniversary gift.

She had been waiting almost seventy years to make that journey and she asked me if I could possibly send her addresses and phone numbers so she could contact the family overseas in advance. My heart was dancing with joy. This was right up my alley. I blew the dust off of my computer and pulled up all of my old genealogy records. It was late, but that didn't matter. I feverishly banged out the information she needed as fast as my fingers would fly. Not only did I find the information she needed, but I was momentarily speechless as I looked at the work I had done those years before. This little assignment reintroduced me to someone I had forgotten about years ago . . . myself. My spirit was coming alive again as I reread parts of the genealogy which I had written when I was researching my family roots. I was touching on those old feelings again.

The girl who wrote that stuff was on a mission. She had a zest for life which few people understood. She wrote well, with a creative energy and an interesting flowery descriptive character which made the dialog informative, yet amusing. On one occasion in particular, flying home after a very special adventure with her Dad, she wrote how she recalled looking down from the sky over Ireland, and it occurred to her that the emerald checker board of the land reminded her of a journey that she would never forget. Her life had changed.

She had changed, blessed, richer from the gift of family connection and kinship with those she had met along the way, and with greater knowledge and respect for those that had gone before her. She recalled reading a passage once and it rang very true. On that day, she discovered, like all those determined searchers who had traced their families back through time . . . and found . . . themselves. That same girl today could barely scrape together a creative thought, nor type so much as something like "See Dick . . . See Dick Run . . . " without struggling.

The next day, I went to visit my own Dad. He still lived in the same old house he had lived in for almost fifty years. His house was only a five minute drive from my own, but I wasn't visiting him the way I should. I had been neglecting him lately but now I was going to deliver the great news of Aunt Mary and her upcoming adventure. I bopped through the door with a spring in my step, and Aunt Mary's letter clutched in my hand. I really enjoyed talking things over with my Dad. My Dad represented so many of the important things in my life. He was a one-of-a-kind character. He was always there for me in good times and in bad, but was always careful about handing out unsolicited advice. When I think of my Dad, I think of the two most precious gifts he gave me in life. He gave me my roots . . . and he gave me my wings.

It would be a nice, refreshing change to share in some good news. He would be thrilled. My smile quickly faded. Dad looked very tired. He had his own declining health issues over the years, but this time he looked worried. He told me he was noticing some weakness in his limbs, tremors in his jaw and hands, and was having dizzy spells. He had a headache in the lower left back section of his head which wasn't going away. He put his hand on the area to show me. He was having trouble walking and negotiating up and down the stairs. I felt a rush of panic as he had suffered through two strokes and a heart attack several of years ago. He told me that he loved me. My Dad, for as much as I had always known that he did, would never say the words "I love you."

Dad would never complain about his own health issues as that was not at all in his nature. Today was different and today he was talking. He quietly explained that these spells weren't actually spells. It seems that he was having trouble with his balance all of the time and this had been going on for a month. He had increased noticeable confusion and his short term memory was really failing. Good God, I know what that means. Dad, like me, would seldom visit a doctor, and usually had to be dragged there against his will.

This time he had made his own appointment. He went to his primary doctor and was scheduled for a MRI the following week. If the results were inconclusive, he was going to a specialist to be tested for Parkinson's Disease. My heart sank. This was one hand which was dealt that I really don't want to play, but life doesn't work that way. There was a large tear in my tapestry. My Dad was in trouble. All I can do is wait.

# XXIX

## "Hello . . . I'm Back! . . . Goodbye . . . I'm Gone"

First Mom, then Walter, and now my own Dad. I can't handle losing another person I love, and I am not ever going to be prepared for the day when my own Dad decides to leave us. Letting go of Walter was going to be a different kind of challenge. I don't really understand it yet, but from the things I was reading, the process would require a certain type of separation where we accept that he is no longer with us per se, yet his body may continue to function for years. I'm not exactly sure how you are expected to ease into this while watching the decline of your loved one, but I guess I will find out soon enough. I decided that if we are ever really going to accept things for what they are, we need to understand the reality of the final third, the advanced or what they call the severe stage. I have been reading the grim details of what to expect next.

We have accepted that we are all now strangers to Dad. Nonetheless, we love him and that is that. David and I dutifully set out to visit Walter. At least we have no more expectations and no longer feel required to come up with riveting conversation. That helps in a way I think, because we are not disappointed anymore. We have lowered that bar right down to the floor now. No expectations, no disappointments, nowhere else to go. Maybe we are giving ourselves credit for personal growth with knowledge and acceptance, when maybe it's just that we are so tired that we are numb. David let out a sigh, punched in the code and we passed through the security doors.

Our silence was abruptly interrupted by something we hadn't heard in quite some time . . . an old, familiar voice. "David, I had a feeling you would be coming to see me today!" Walter said in a complete unbroken sentence. David and I stopped dead in our tracks as we stared at Dad. Walter was just kind of standing there with a smile on his face. Dad knew David . . . he knew his name and who he was, his son. This was only the beginning. We walked down the hall with him and Walter actually read his own name plate on his door. He read the "Drilling & Blasting" sign in his shadow box and even recognized his own First Holy Communion picture.

He pointed at the photo of his stock car and began to tell us about the old days. He told us all about growing up and visiting his cousin who lived several towns away. This cousin became a car enthusiast and had a wonderful vintage car collection. Walter went on to describe how he and Anne went to visit him many years later and he still had all of his wonderful cars. He went on to describe the old Packards, and even his cousin's prize Tucker.

It was incredible, the details were all correct. It was just incredible. I am confused. We lose Walter because specific areas of the brain have been affected by the disease. Then he is back again. So what is actually going on in there? One doctor had said, "Alzheimer's doesn't move smoothly from one stage of the disease to the next. Life becomes a series of jumps and starts—two steps forward, one step back. You can expect to experience sadness, depression, anger, resignation, even acceptance over and over again."

Okay, so he still doesn't recognize me, but today he is just unbelievable. I'm taking this man to Wal-Mart next time and I'm putting him in charge of my cart. He is just great! He is perfect! I listened to myself, and thought of the hundreds of times I wanted to reach out and strangle those well-wishing visitors that would tell me those exact words. Days like this are a mixed blessing for me. This is the hardest part, the acceptance part of Alzheimer's. You struggle and struggle with letting go, you finally come to certain terms and make yourself accept things for what they are as the disease marches on.

Then one day you walk in, finally comfortable with this new level of understanding. It has taken you months, by the way, months to accept this new comfort level, and then he has a day like today. What has happened? What is going on? Does this have anything to do with the medication? Is he getting better? Was this all just a big misunderstanding? Now a million questions begin to whirl around in our heads. The cruel reality of this disease is that quite randomly, it can quickly restore everyone's hope. And in a flash, the hope is torn away again. In a moment, we are all strangers again. Back to the way it was before, only we are more confused and a little shaken because we know good old Dad is in there somewhere, trapped inside of himself, just like the doctor had said.

This kind of thing began to happen more frequently. Walter was here . . . Walter was gone . . . Walter was here . . . Walter was gone. When Walter made an appearance, it was more like having a really great dream. You know what I mean, the kind of dream where you are really enjoying yourself and everyone is happy, when suddenly you are woken up abruptly. You are a little confused while you momentarily decide if it was real or not. It was not real, it was only a dream. You want to close your eyes and resume the dream again. You want to pick up right where you left off. But that never works. Instead you drag yourself out of bed and face reality.

Our next visit with Dad reminded us again of just how this disease can be so cruel. Dad was gone again, still quite cheerful but lost in his own little world. Today we were all strangers. David found Walter and Patrick down in the community room. David suggested that they take a stroll outside in the garden area and the two men maneuvered off of the couch with enthusiasm. They were more than willing to go on any small adventure with David. I just wanted to sit quietly. I picked out a little corner table in the vacant bistro area where we had Walter's birthday party several months earlier. Sometimes I just liked to watch the residents come and go. I liked to watch how they interacted with the staff, with their visitors and with each other. It was still all quite interesting to me.

I noticed some of my old friends go by, but I didn't call out to them and they didn't seem to notice me. I saw some new faces too, and I found myself letting out a long, slow sigh as I studied each face. I recognized the far away image of that familiar small frame, sporting the pink sweater set and clutching the matching purse. It was Katie, and she was making her way down the hall toward me. She seemed confused and was checking each room along the way as if she was looking for someone. She must be frantically searching for Patrick and Walter. She probably didn't see them go out into the courtyard garden with David, and now she must be worried.

I got up to greet her and I was prepared to ease her concern by telling her where her two men were. As I started to explain, I could see that she was very agitated. She wasn't listening and was instead searching up and down each corridor with her eyes. She almost looked frantic. I stopped talking and looked at her face. Something was very wrong. She began asking if I had seen her son, Mike. She said he was supposed to be here and she can't find him. I remembered what he looked like from his photos, although they were older photos, and I told her I would watch out for him. She seemed a little relieved, but continued her frantic search down the hall. I sat back down and began to think. I have come to recognize that thinking was bad. I really don't need to be thinking every little thing over. When it comes to these issues, I think it all over to death. Then I rehash it again . . . just for fun.

Actually, I was really hoping that her son, Mike would come for a visit today. I had been wanting to meet him for many months now. I sat up straight and began to watch the access door, listening for the familiar click sound it would make as a visitor would punch in the correct access code. I wanted to tell him what really wonderful parents he had. I wanted to tell him about the cute things his Dad did, and about his Mom showing me her "booby-trap" door alarm. I was going to ask David if we could stay a while longer today. I thought that I might just be able to say a couple of things to Mike that would make him feel just a little bit better about having both his parents here.

I watched for a long time and then started becoming agitated myself. Where was he? Didn't he know his poor mother was frantically searching for him? Did something more important come up and now he's not coming? Maybe he was some big corporate somebody and work was more important. Did he always do this kind of thing to her? I was actually getting angry, as I could still see Katie's far away figure down the hall, going in and out of each room. She asked the passing staff members if they had seen Mike, and they either just silently shook their heads, or they answered, "No, Katie, I don't think he is coming today." I let out a disgruntled huff. They didn't care, and how did they know he wasn't coming anyway? Couldn't they have just taken an extra moment to say something encouraging to her. Any idiot could see she was upset. What was wrong with these people anyway?

I saw Elizabeth passing by. Elizabeth was the wife of Edward, that very young resident with Alzheimer's. Elizabeth was that very nice woman who had spent a lot of time at the facility and she knew a lot about the residents. She also knew a lot about their families too. She helped us with encouraging words when we first brought Dad here. She had watched out for Dad. She took a special interest in the lives of these people, and she was a caring person. She would know the scoop on Mike's whereabouts.

Elizabeth stopped for a minute and we exchanged pleasantries. We talked about Walter and Edward for a minute. She always reminded me of what a sweet and nice man Walter was. Then I decided to ask her if Katie and Patrick had any visitors lately. She thought for a moment and proceeded to tell me that the only visitor she had ever seen was a niece. She had talked to the niece when Katie and Patrick had first arrived and Elizabeth said she had only seen her a couple of times over the months as she believed the niece lived out of state. She thought that the niece was in charge of their affairs and brought them clothes from time to time.

She could see the confused and somewhat agitated look on my face and asked me what was wrong. Elizabeth must have been mistaken . . . I knew she wasn't. I was afraid to ask, but I finally choked out the words. I said, "What about their son, their son Mike?" She looked at me for a long while before she slowly answered me. "Mike . . . " she said, "I'm pretty sure that was the name of their only child. The niece had told me that Mike had died. He had died in an auto accident." I gasped as she continued, "He was only in his mid-thirties at the time when the accident happened . . . more than twenty five years ago."

# XXX
## Not Such a Beautiful Sunset

For a long time now, I had avoided more reading about the final or third stage of Alzheimer's Disease. More statistics and clinical research offer explanations but understanding does not change the outcome. There is no cure. Still, some of these mounds of documentation may help me to accept things and move on. In a nutshell, this is what I learned about what is going on in Walter's body.

I have learned that he has lower levels of acetylcholine in certain areas of the brain. This is the chemical messenger, or neurotransmitter needed for the brain cells to work properly. The article talked about senile plaques, which are clumps of abnormal nerve cells surrounding abnormal protein deposits and neurofibrillary tangles. These tangles are the material that disrupt the normal structure of nerve cells.

These brain changes cause memory loss and decline of all other mental abilities. Eventually the changes affect functional and physical abilities and would lead to eventual death. It was not possible to measure the progress of the disease as the extent of senile plaques and neurofibrillary tangles can only be determined after death through autopsy. I paused and put down the book.

Did I really need to know all of this? All of this was hardly gripping stuff and I hesitated to read on. Something told me to stop denying the grim sequence of events and to simply accept the path which was chosen. It seemed as if this story was not really about Walter after all. It was about challenges presented to me, and how I would choose to meet these challenges. I opted to keep on reading.

Walter had now passed through the second or moderate stage. I recognized each and every symptom and my mind recalled exact examples of what the documentation had described. I recall many instances of him having difficulties recognizing close friends and family members. He had become restless at times, wandering and confused especially in the late afternoon and evening hours. The books refer to this as "Sundowning." He had problems reading, writing and dealing with numbers. He had trouble organizing his thoughts and thinking logically. Many times he struggled with finding the right words to say, and he would make up stories to fill in the blanks. He had lost all recognition of time. He no longer knew what year, what month, what day it was, or even if it were morning, noon or night.

Walter had trouble dressing, and now needs continuous assistance. He gets upset easily and at times has had short outbursts with the staff. Once in a while he becomes a little hostile and is unwilling to cooperate with them, although he can't really communicate what is bothering him. The staff was taken by surprise the first time this happened as this behavior was not at all in his character. As an aide was describing his new behavior, I secretly wondered if maybe he was getting sick and tired of having his shoes jammed on the wrong feet.

At times, especially when he first arrived at the facility, he expressed firmly held false beliefs or delusions, suspicion of others and agitation. He would frantically describe how people were moving his furniture at night. He described how they took his furniture away and had refinished it, returning it the next morning. He told us they were doing that every night. He said they had done a good job (still always a kind word), but that he did not ask them to do it and he worried about paying for it. He would run his hand over his dresser to show us all the work they did. I would frantically search every inch of the wood finish with my eyes, looking for any little small sign or detail that would prove his story just might have been true.

There was a time, not so long ago where I had only read about those signs of disease progression, and now I am looking back on them like they were a fulfilled prophecy. Walter passed through the first and second stage with textbook accuracy. I am now starting to recognize the very early signs of the third and final stage. He is not there yet but he has already touched on the first signs of phase three. Walter can no longer remember how to bathe, eat, dress or go to the bathroom independently. This has been going on for a while.

As I had said before, I am no longer focused on lowering the bar of acceptance with every new small indication of decline, convincing myself that this "isn't so bad." I am past the denial stage. It is bad. There seems to be no more good that I can squeak out of an incident or situation that I can see. I am always still looking for a tiny gift from God though, a moment when that warm and wonderful man will make a small appearance. Any small sign that he is still with us.

And so the article read . . . . Walter may become even more confused near the evening and the condition known as "Sundowning" will become more evident. He will have increased difficulty sleeping. Walter will have trouble walking and may fall frequently. He may become confined to a wheelchair or become bedridden as eventually he will be unable to control the movement of his muscles. He will eventually lose the ability to chew and swallow his food. His food will have to be ground and he will need to be fed. At some point, he will no longer be able to communicate with words and will completely lose bladder and bowel control.

During the late phase with his struggle with Alzheimer's Disease, Walter may become more vulnerable to other illnesses. Occasionally, people with the disease will experience seizures. Death often occurs from complications of being confined to a bed, such as contracting pneumonia. The article was meant as a tool to prepare the care giver, family and friends for the end. It described the physical and emotional changes which occur as death approaches. I remembered the sequence of events which occurred when Mom died, and this article touched on each sign with precision. Walter was always one who believed in sticking to the rules, and something tells me he will do just that until the end.

The rules say that Walter will develop excessive sleepiness and weakness as his overall energy declines. His breathing will change with rapid breathing alternated with short episodes when breathing stops. His visual and hearing changes also. He may see people or places that others do not. I flashed back to the night when Anne tried to show me the beautiful angel by her bed. Grandma, Walter's mother, tried to show me her departed sister right before she left us too. The rules went on to say that Walter will have a decreased appetite. As his metabolism slows, he will no longer be interested in food. His urinary and bowel functions will change. His urine may become dark or red.

Walter's body temperature may begin to fluctuate, high one moment and very cold the next. I saw all of these signs years ago when I had worked for the nursing home as well as when Anne died. There will be emotional changes as well as Walter will begin the separation process. He will become less interested in the outside world, socially separating himself from loved ones, or people who as care givers had become his friends on whatever level of recognition he will have with each of them when the time comes. Finally he will let go.

I sat quietly and thought about what I had just read. Did I feel any better about anything, knowing the grim reality about Walter's future? I don't think so. I don't think I felt worse though either, as I already knew what was in store for him if he lived long enough. I guess I was just hoping he didn't have to carry it out all the way to the awful end as the books describe. It's all out of our hands anyway, and whatever way is chosen, was meant for a reason. Walter will follow the rules and will do as he is told. I think of myself when someday it will be my turn, and I smile just a tiny smile as I know I will probably be battling the rules until the end, refusing to "go toward the light" as God is instructing me to do so, arguing that I'd rather do it my own way.

The article about death taught me a few more things about life. It said that grief is a normal and healthy reaction which often takes two years or more to go through the most intense emotions of the grieving process. Although the sense of loss may never go away, we all just need time to come to terms with the normal shock, denial, anger and guilt that is often felt by the ones left behind after losing a loved one. Each person must come to terms with the loss in their own individual way. I really understand that now.

It occurred to me that perhaps we never properly allowed ourselves to grieve for Mom as we were immediately thrown into the mayhem of caring for Dad. Confusion was a part of our everyday life as we dealt with the enormous responsibilities that went along with being a care giver. In fact, I know we didn't allow ourselves any time or room for grieving. Everything else, including her death was put on the back burner to be dealt with later. There was never really the time to think about how we were all feeling because our lives had changed so dramatically almost overnight. We never ever dealt with what was on the back burner.

And so the article said . . . In the past, death was visible and dealt with openly. A dying person was almost always cared for at home. My grandparents spoke of this very thing as they took care of their parents back in the old country. Advances in medical technology had made death more removed from everyday life. People near the end of life are now most often cared for in hospitals or nursing homes. As a result, many people are less familiar and less comfortable with the dying process. Aggressive medical interventions have prolonged life, even in the face of long term illness. As a result, some may view the illness as conquerable and view death as something that can and should be avoided as long as possible, at any cost and without regard to quality of life . . . Wow, was this article written just for me, or what?

With every step along the way, I seemed to be doing battle with something completely out of my control, frantically trying to find answers and a way out with a happy ending for Walter. It seems that I am in control of nothing when to comes to helping Walter along his path, except for just being there for him in whatever capacity he needs me, a friend, a stranger or just the chocolate lady. It doesn't matter what I think I can do next as Walter will find his own gentle, almost organized, natural and personal way through this.

I am letting go of a lot of old feelings lately. They were feelings of anger and frustration, insensitivity at times and feelings of neglect for Walter at times. Letting go feels good. I do not feel shame as I once did with these thoughts. A doctor had once written "From the moment someone is diagnosed with Alzheimer's, there are always at least two who are diagnosed as the lives closest to him will never be the same." This is so very true and is tough stuff to handle, but the bottom line now is that Walter and the other residents are being well taken care of. The rest is up to God.

In reality, I am extremely sensitive to all of my new resident friends afflicted with this horrible disease. I have learned so much about myself. I have amazing respect and even love for these people who don't even know me. I have learned not to judge other people, and I have learned that everyone I meet is at some point in their life, going to have to face some kind of life altering challenge and they too will need to dig down deep to find, within themselves, what they are really made of. When it comes to Walter, I need to be willing to accept whatever comes next, and maybe I can do it with just a little more grace and dignity than I have done in the past. Thanks for that lesson, Walter.

Well, with all that being said, I feel much better. It all sounds so simple, yet the underlying most destructive demon in this whole thing is a story about depression. Of course we have all heard about it, but I was much too smart, much too strong and much too busy to give something like that a moment of my precious time. I was not really all that smart after all. I was doing some real damage there. God forbid I should dare to type in "Depression" on my web search, because if I was having a problem with this, it was surely something that was within my control. I have been feeling sad and hopeless for a long time now, I'm sure it's nothing. Well . . . being that there is nothing good on TV, maybe I'll just pull up a website and see what the experts have to say.

"Depression—A mood disorder that causes you to feel sad or hopeless for an extended period of time. Depression can have a significant impact on your enjoyment of life, your work, your health and the people you care about."

Okay, so maybe some people have that, but I think for them, it may be more a case of a personal weakness, or a character flaw. There can't be any real medical basis for depression. Regular people like me should be strong enough to just pull out of it on their own. Gosh, I am smart, but maybe I'll just read a little more.

"People with depression may be reluctant to seek help because they feel that it is a sign of personal weakness, a character flaw or that they should just be able to pull out of it on their own. We now know that depression, like other medical conditions, has a chemical and biological basis. Treatment for depression is safe and usually effective even for severely depressed people."

I still think I have all of the answers, but something made me keep reading. The article said that depression is triggered by stressful life events, other illnesses, certain drugs, medications or inherited traits. Symptoms included a depressed mood, inability to enjoy activities, problems concentrating, memory deficiencies, difficulty making decisions, changes in eating habits, and weight gain or loss.

The article continued . . . . Difficulty focusing on taking care of daily responsibilities, feelings of guilt, slowed thoughts and speech and complaints which have no apparent physical cause, such as headaches and stomachaches. So far, this author has pretty much summed up the past few years of my life. With the exception of not actually posting my photograph with the article, the article was certainly all about me.

The article stated that a health professional usually successfully treats depression with counseling and antidepressant medication. Those were exactly the words I did not want to read. The only pill I want to put down my throat is my Flintstone Vitamin each morning. I continued reading, nonetheless. Here's what I learned. I was not alone. In the United States, fifteen percent of all people will have depression at some point in life, most commonly between the ages of twenty-five and forty-five. The article stated that it was important to break the cycle of depression. If not recognized and treated, one would run the risk of more severe depression or becoming physically ill. Sounds like my old friend, the ''loop'' thing again.

The author discussed Cognitive Behavior Therapy. It's a type of counseling that focuses on modifying certain thoughts and behavior patterns to control the symptoms of a condition. Cognitive Behavior Therapy is used to treat a variety of problems, including stress, depression, anxiety, panic disorders, eating disorders, chronic pain and chronic fatigue syndrome. Nineteen million Americans are feeling just like me, and I thought I was all alone.

I think I just may reach out and talk to someone. I think it could help me, but he or she had better not try to suggest medication with me. I know that it has worked wonders for many people, and I respect any and all things those people have done to help themselves. Sadly, it is clear that I don't know everything and once or twice I have been wrong in my life, but I just don't want to go that medication route. I wanted to be free, but not that way. That was just not me.

Talking would be a good thing. I chuckled as I imagined the stunned and forlorn look upon the face of my would-be counselor as I opened my mouth and began to unload years of pent-up frustrations. I am sure that they have heard it all. Still, a part of me says that I got myself into this and I could jolly well get myself back out. Life is what you make of it. It was true, that riding along with Walter on his journey was probably the most difficult challenge I had been handed so far in my life. I had never experienced anything which had touched me so deeply or in so many ways. I had never felt so out of control or defeated sometimes. I also believed what I had said in the beginning, that each of life's experiences, both good and bad, changes who you are just a little.

Maybe I was aware of that all along and maybe I didn't want to change. Maybe I was wallowing in some self-pity, some of which was my own making. Just reading the testimonials of others who were struggling had helped me immensely and I could feel that fighting spirit coming alive again. A well-meaning friend of mine suggested that I should go on vacation, maybe back to Ireland to reconnect with my family. That would be a nice thing, but first things first. I know that my pot of gold is not to be found in County Kerry, it is to be found deep inside of myself.

# XXXI
## Unfinished Business

I had some very important unfinished business to take care of. I had decided that it was important to me to go and have a little talk with Mom. I knew it was going to take a while to get a few things off of my chest so I brought a large cup of hot coffee, my warmest jacket, and a big box of Kleenex. I drove up to the cemetery by myself and sat on the ground in front of her stone. I studied the stone for a while as I prepared my speech. You see, it was a little tricky. I was angry with her. After all of these years, I was still angry but would never dare to admit this to anyone. I had issues that went back many years but with the news of her illness, I decided to sweep it all under the carpet.

We had done a lot of things with Mom and Dad over the years. We took trips and vacations together, went out to breakfast and dinner several times a week together. We went on drives every Sunday afternoon together, and visited them every day in between. My issue had always been that Anne was not always kind to me. I thought I had made peace with her in the end, but the truth was, I hadn't. If I had told anyone how I was feeling, I felt they would have told me to just get over it. After all, what kind of a frightful human being would I have been, uttering unpleasantness to a dying woman. My issues may have sounded petty in light of everything else that was going on and so I kept it all safely tucked away.

I looked at her stone for a long time, still bothered that she didn't get her pink granite with the engraved heart. I looked at Walter's name carved into the granite above hers. His birth date was already engraved and I stared at the blank spot where his date of death would someday be. I wondered what it would read. I drew a deep breath and began. I told her that I was not angry that she had kept so many things a secret, especially about Walter. I told her that I understood that she was from the old school where you kept the family secrets carefully guarded.

I had also come to realize that although it may have been helpful for us to have known what was really going on, I'm not sure we would have conducted ourselves any differently. Time had taught me that our delusions of following that "well-thought-out plan" did not ever work out for us at any stage of the disease. Most things had to be worked out the hard way as we went along.

I was angry for things now, things that I didn't clearly understand years ago. Anne and Walter enjoyed life. That was good, but I felt that they enjoyed it sometimes at other's expense. I remembered how they loved to travel with their friends, and spent many months away from home each year in Florida. I recalled how when Walter's parents were very old and his father was ill, they left as scheduled for their three months in warm paradise. We begged them not to go that year. The care-giving responsibilities were thrust upon Joan. I could not fully appreciate what that was like until now, but I knew at the time that it wasn't right.

I remember placing several unreturned phone calls to them as Grandpa was dying. When they did call, it was to recount their adventures and describe how wonderful it was down there. We begged them to come home and at one point Anne indignantly announced that "It's our vacation." We had to insist that they return as the end was near. They spent time with Grandma and Grandpa when things were fine, but I felt that they did not pitch in when times were bad. They were always gone. Nothing was going to get in the way of their plans . . . nothing.

I was also angry because they dumped their business affairs upon David while they were gone, leaving him in charge of unresolved legal affairs and keeping their appointments time after time. Anne would again indignantly tell us that this was their retirement, and they were going to enjoy it. I recalled being annoyed because since the time in their lives that they were our age, they were flying to all kinds of wonderful destinations and were enjoying life.

I had nothing against any of that but I felt that if you're going to do that, you can at least have all of your own affairs taken care of first. I felt that it didn't bother them that they were being selfish with other people's time. It was simply understood that David would jump in there and take care of it all every time they left. The responsibilities never seemed to be doled out to anyone else. That was how they ran their lives and they thought nothing of it. I took exception to the whole routine, as I was now a part of it.

I was aggravated by their house too. Every inch of the place, every drawer, cupboard, closet, nook and cranny was filled with old junk and papers it seemed. Every time I needed to open a drawer it was jammed shut as it was full of all kinds of miscellaneous oddities. Every time I needed to open a cupboard, fifty years worth of old dented tin foil TV dinner trays, and old deformed plastic Cool Whip containers would fall on my head. They had been missing their lids for years and were never used. David was forever searching for something important, in despair and with great mounds of stuff everywhere. We had asked them so many times if we could start cleaning out the upstairs bedrooms, which were packed to the ceiling with old broken stuff. The answer was always an indignant "No!" How dare we even have the nerve to mention that they part with their stuff.

There again, you can't go around telling others how to live. I certainly wouldn't like it. To each his own and I respect that. The problem had more to do with the fact that we knew this would be thrust upon us one day. Rather selfish thinking on our part? No, maybe years ago it would have been none of our business. It was my opinion that they had made it our business by again assuming it would just be our responsibility to deal with it all later. I learned something from this. I knew how it felt, and I organized all of my affairs and threw away boxes of old stuff piled up in my own basement and attic. It was nice to feel organized, and it will someday be a way to say "I love you" to the poor person who will be in charge of our affairs when we can no longer handle things for ourselves.

We became concerned as they were getting older too. David had built some safety railings for the entrance to their house. We were concerned about the access to their bathroom. Their bathroom was very narrow and not up to any kind of code. It was hard for a person in good shape to maneuver sideways past the sink and tub to get to the toilet. Turning around in there was a challenge. If one of them ever had to use a cane or walker, they would have never been able to get around in there. There was a walk-in closet adjoining the bathroom. It was almost never used, except as another place to pile up more old junk. David approached them with a plan to knock out the wall between the bathroom and the closet, and expand the bathroom over an extra six feet so at least it would be accessible in the future. He offered to do the work himself.

They both immediately dismissed the idea, clearly stating that no one . . . no one was going to tell them what to do. They were taking their money and they were going on vacation instead. When Anne became ill, that little bathroom became hell for us all. She could not go in there alone in the end, because she needed a walker and it would not fit in there. It was also too small for two people. Not only could we not assist her to the toilet, but getting her and her shower chair in and out of the tub was another challenge. Through the years, she always dug her heels in deeper and remained stubbornly steadfast when it came to any kind of compromise. She did not like it if we asked something of them. What we were asking was always for their benefit and for no other reason.

I suppose I should have been aggravated with Walter as well, as he was always silently standing by as these things were happening. I wasn't. I'm not sure exactly why but I always held him blameless over the years, regardless of the conflict. I could always see through to the inside of his most kind soul. He would silently walk away instead of being dragged into any kind of altercation. Sometimes, it seemed to me, he was just doing as he was told. He had to see what some of these things were doing to us, but I don't remember him ever stepping in. Walter was just Walter, that was his way and I loved him for exactly who he was. Period.

I was angry at Anne for other reasons too. Holidays were always torture. I had always loved the holidays, but I had grown to dislike them. She would always tell me weeks in advance how much trouble the holidays were and how other family member's daughters-in-law would clean their houses for them. She would tell me how "they would do this . . . they would do that . . . " She complained about shopping. She complained about wrapping. She would say that she didn't have time for any of it.

Even when Jackie and his family were coming up from Florida, she would never prepare their rooms or even put up a Christmas tree. It was always the same. The complaining

185

started months in advance and then the night before they flew in, David and I were frantically cleaning her house, making their beds and putting up the Christmas tree to perpetuate the illusion of a good ole fashioned New England Christmas for the rest of the family.

We had obligations with other family members during the holidays too and always asked Anne for consideration when it came to planning meal time so we could plan visits with others as well. Never once would she bend. Other family member's plans and dinners would just have to wait. One Christmas in particular was very sad for me, as my cousin was very ill with cancer. He was just two months younger than I was and it had been an awful year for him and the rest of the family. The call came on Christmas Eve. He was given last rites. It was an empty holiday for me. My heart was just not into having a Merry Christmas.

I can only remember sitting at the dinner table, shocked as Anne was spitting out my casserole, literally spitting it out on her plate and barking "what did you put in this anyway?" Walter and David froze. The two of them with that "deer in the headlights" stunned gaze. They both quickly looked at me and then looked down at their plates and continued on eating as if nothing were wrong. No one said a word. No one defended me. I quietly imagined what she would have looked like with her plate of food dumped upon her festive new hair-do. It was yet another frosty Silent Night.

As I sat with my eyes fixed on her stone, I asked Anne why twenty years ago when it was just two weeks before our wedding, she announced that they were going to Maine to go fishing, and they were not sure if they would be back in time. I asked her why we had to reschedule the rehearsal dinner at my Dad's house because she wouldn't tell us one way or the other if they would be there. Apparently, that time of the month was when "the ice was going out on the lake in Maine and that's when they liked to go fishing."

Our wedding had been planned for months and she had never said a word about any of that. Not until two freaking weeks before the big event. David did not say a word. We all walked on eggshells some more, wondering what the outcome would be. Oh. P.S., she didn't like my wedding dress either. We pressed on. The whole thing put a cloud of sadness over the weeks which lead up to our wedding day. It was supposed to be a time of joy and excitement and she took that away from me. She knew she did, and I knew that she knew. We kept up appearances as usual and she showed up on time in her new dress with smiles for everyone and for the cameras. It was a cycle which continued for twenty years.

The coolness accelerated when we bought our house. This now put the distance between us to nine miles. After years of living only a few hundred feet from them, it was now nine precious miles. They would visit us occasionally at first, and then they stopped. It was too far she said, yet they could jump in the black Buick and drive for hours to go to lunch at the shore. She would still think nothing of calling David all hours of the night and day to drive over and attend to emergencies, like to loosen the lid on the mayonnaise jar. When they would visit, she would remark "Aren't you lucky to always have new things," or "Isn't it nice to have someone to always buy you things." Luck had very little to do with the fact that I had worked very hard for many years to pay for whatever I owned, and where was this "someone" who was buying me this stuff, anyway? I always bought and paid for my own stuff. Did I miss something?

She knew how hard I worked, and she did not approve of the fact that I spent a lot of time away from home. I was always going to school as part of my work, or was away at training seminars. She always came up just short of saying that I was not good enough for her son. Other people would tell me that Anne would say nice things about me yet I never actually heard anything like that myself. I never understood her, and she never understood me. I only knew that she was the cause of rifts between myself and David. Just once I would have liked him to stand up for me. Maybe if I had stood up for myself years ago, things would have been much different. Maybe I wouldn't be getting frostbite in this cemetery right now.

I recalled how there was yet another very cool breeze in the air on one sunny Sunday afternoon. We had invited them over for lunch on the new deck we had just built. I had worked for hours preparing salads and desserts, dips and drinks, baked chicken and fresh vegetables. Everything was arranged and prepared. The table was set. They only had to sit down. I couldn't sit down. There was apparently something wrong with everything I had made. She wanted this instead . . . she wanted that instead . . . this didn't taste right . . . that didn't taste right . . . .

Walter and David ate silently as I jumped up and down obeying each command to get her something else. This went on for quite some time. This was not right. I had really put a lot of time and effort into preparing the meal. Everyone else was almost done and I hadn't even started. This type of thing had happened on many occasions before, but this time she was treating me like this in my own home. She had gone too far. I looked over at my two big strong men for a little support. Nothing . . . . I got nothing.

I finally sat down once more when she announced that the water now tasted funny. It had been fine two minutes ago, but now it tasted funny. I remember silently, and with no facial expression at all, just reaching across the table, picking up her glass, and hurling the contents directly over my head, over the deck railing to the ground below. I gently and silently replaced the now empty glass down in front of her and kept on eating. Now I had three "deer in the headlights" gazes staring at me. Just as I could have predicted, all faces in unison silently looked down at their plates and continued eating. My ears were going to be burning that night as I knew that Walter was going to suffer the wrath for every one of those very long nine miles back to their home. Just in case anyone was interested, I felt perfectly fine. No . . . I felt great.

I was further annoyed because of her refusal to get a hearing aid. It was all about vanity, the stigma, the social unacceptability, worry of what others would say. It became very exasperating for the rest of us when it came to day to day communication with her. She could hear very little, almost nothing unless you screamed at her over and over again. Three times for each occurrence was my limit. I would try to say something to her, each time raising my voice until I was actually yelling. If she didn't get it by the third yell, I would simply stop and look at David. It would be up to him to yell louder until the message got across. It was very stressful attempting that kind of communication all of the time. I could always feel my blood pressure going up until I could actually feel the blood pounding in my head.

Although we tried to show her advertisements of hearing aids, she refused to consider them even though they were quite tiny and would go undetected, especially with her hair styled the way she did. She was still convinced that they were as they were years ago, with a box that hung down and wires tangled. We tried to tell her that it was nothing to be ashamed of, and nobody would know anyway unless she wanted to tell them. Even if they did know . . . so what? What was wrong with having one? In the meantime, it was making us all crazy. She didn't seem to care about that.

I was never the saintly daughter-in-law, but I had tried my best. As a matter of fact, I felt I had gone far beyond the call of duty to keep harmony over the years. I didn't want to alienate myself from the rest of the family as I loved them all. Anne had this way of always needing to show me that she had a certain control over David. I thought it was stupid, and a waste of energy. I would become annoyed with her frequent stories which always started with "Poor Ray . . . " or "Poor Jackie . . ." Please, give me a break. I didn't want thanks or praise for all of the times we had been there for them, but I didn't want to hear "Poor Ray . . . " or "Poor Jackie" anymore. Nothing really ever changed much in the routine of Anne and Walter. They continued on their vacations as usual, leaving David in various dilemmas with their affairs. His own work would wait.

The events leading up to Anne's death were interesting to me and were clearly a favor to us from God. You see, four months before Anne left us, she actually died . . . twice. One night, she had a heart attack and was rushed to the emergency room by ambulance. By the time we arrived, we were told that her heart had stopped twice for a period of time before they were able to get it restarted again. Thanks to the great emergency staff and the defibrillator, she had somehow pulled through. She had burns on her chest and had no recollection of that missing time frame. She remained in the hospital for about a week while they ran a battery of tests. They eventually said she could go home and recover there.

We were emotionally traumatized over the whole ordeal but were ready to step in and nurse her back to health. Not only could we do it, but we were going to do it better than anyone else. It wasn't until a few weeks later, when she was getting weaker instead of better, that the doctors decided to run some more tests. They found advanced liver and pancreatic cancer. We were stunned. How could they have missed this whole terrible thing when she was in the hospital for the heart attack? She was having tests and blood work done the whole time, and a multitude of medically advanced testing of all sorts done daily. How was it even possible that this whole thing went totally undetected?

Here was the odd thing about our relationship. I thought it could never change, but it did in some ways, and very quickly. I remember very well that day that I walked into their living room as Anne, Walter and David sat quietly on the couch.

"What's wrong?" I said as I studied their faces. David proceeded to tell me about Anne's test results and that her condition was terminal. She was told she had about four to six months to live. I was shocked. I remembered bending down and giving her a hug. I told her I was sorry. This was a family that never hugged each other, well, maybe on a holiday, but that was always awkward. I was truly sorry. I didn't want her to suffer. I wouldn't want anyone one to die in such a horrible way. All of my many gripes with her over the years seemed quite petty and faded away in an instant. I was now only hoping for enough time to make things right with her. I wasn't sure how, but I was going to try.

I often wondered what had gone on that night in the emergency room when her heart was stopped for a period of time. There was a period of a few minutes where I believe, God was looking down at the sorry bunch of us and decided not to take her just then. He was going to give her and all of us a little more time to prepare and get organized. We needed a little time to prepare Walter slowly. We needed to hear Anne's requests and final wishes. We needed a little time to get her affairs in order and to have her tell us some of the details of their affairs. Dad no longer knew what was going on with any of it.

God knew about Anne's secret of protecting Walter. God knew that Anne was doing most of the day-to-day management of Walter's routine, and that Walter had no clue. God also saw that the rest of us were also walking around with no idea of the overwhelming responsibility that was about to be thrust upon us. I can only assume that he let out a little sigh, shook his head, and sent Anne back for a short time to help us all get organized.

Now that these years have passed, all of the conflicts with Anne seemed childish. As I now sat in the cemetery, I told Anne they were very real to me at the time and I remembered being hurt. I told her that I never was able to just let things go because I had spent so many years choking it all down instead of airing it all out. I told her that I was sorry for the both of us for wasting our time playing that hurtful little game, or whatever it was for all of those years. I told her I was mad at her because she should have been happy that David found someone like me who loved him so much. I told her that I was a hard worker, a good and caring person and I was angry at her for never noticing that. Instead, there was turmoil because she never thought twice about being so demanding with David's time.

I told her I was mad at him too for never once defending his wife against his mother's daggers, instead choosing to look the other way. He was a great son, everyone knew that. He was a good person, everyone knew that too. I told her I was angry because I felt that she sometimes put him into positions in which he would have to choose his wife over his mother, knowing full well that he would not. I told her that after everything I had done to try to fit into the family, that she, in her sometimes not so subtle ways made me feel like I did not. I told her that I was angry at her for making someone like me make promises that were beyond my control. I told her I was angry at myself because I thought it was better under the circumstances to not talk about it in the end and just let it all pass.

I told her that doing that was wrong because I was the one who was still here, sorting out life's lessons, struggling with old hurt and struggling with old guilt. I told her that I had plenty of new hurt and guilt to deal with and that I needed to let go of the old. I must have talked for a good hour or two, until I felt like I had said all of the things I needed to but never dared to say. I secretly wondered if she would have been nicer to me all those years if she knew I was to be her caregiver in the end. I secretly wondered if I had waited until after she was gone before I finally spoke up so I would be able to have the last word.

Wow. . . . Where did all of that come from? I wondered why I had felt it was so important to hash things out with a poor dead woman after all of these years. It seemed clear to me now. I no longer wanted to blame her for many of the hurt feelings I had buried down deep all this time. I had allowed a lot of the unresolved issues to fester for a long time, and her sudden illness seemed to put the more important issues to the front. Forgetting petty differences seemed like the right thing to do at the time. The truth was, the hurtful things which I was harboring really played a significant role in the way I was handling some of the issues with Walter and with life in general. I always felt I could just deal with it. And I did, I guess until we were faced with a multitude of responsibility, endless challenges and sadness all at once, and for a continuous long period of time.

These long ago issues with her confused me. I supposed they were always in the background simmering away unnoticed on the back burner. I was struggling with "trying to be a good person" near her end when what I really wanted to do was to open up, really open up, let it all out and release all of this pent up baggage. I needed closure so I could move on and be able to face even more challenges which would be ahead of me without any old unfinished business in the shadows.

I take responsibility for most of it. One can't simply go around blaming, complaining and wishing they could change other people's behavior. They are who they are. I could have changed the way I allowed other people to affect me though. If things were bothering me, I should have spoken up and not silently allowed incidents to tear me down the way they did. I was now convinced that if I am ever faced with this type of conflict again, I will do better.

Simply saying all of those unpleasant things out loud was a huge relief. My eyes quickly scanned the cemetery again. I certainly didn't want any witnesses to this whole thing. It was a small town. Everybody knew everybody. Come to think of it, they would probably look upon me with admiration, praising me for being such a good daughter-in-law. Ha! . . . little would they know that I was giving a poor dead woman a verbal thrashing for the sake of my own sanity. I blew my nose, took a deep breath and I told her that despite all of the things that had happened, that I had loved her.

Then I told her that I always thought she was a very beautiful woman. I told her that she was a very strong woman and I how I was still amazed at the strength and courage she showed us all right up until the end. I thanked her for choosing me to carry out "Promise Number Two." That in itself told me that she trusted and cared for me. It was her last unexpected and very special gift to me which I will always remember and cherish. I told her that I admired the deep love that she shared with Walter for all of those years.

I sat quietly looking at her stone again, waiting for an answer. There was no booming voice from the sky. There was no giant lightning bolt either. That was good. What I felt instead was very gentle. I had a feeling, a comforting feeling of understanding from or for Anne. I'm not sure which and I decided it was both. It seemed to go both ways. I think she was faced with sorting it all out on the night she went to meet her maker a long time ago. I think she saw things from a much more enlightened perspective once she got to her destination. I felt that wherever she was, she was sorry for the way she sometimes treated me. I felt that she appreciated me now where she may not have before. I felt that she loved me. I felt she was watching me, and was helping me as she promised. I felt she was watching us all from a distance as we helped Walter. I felt that she was feeling all of our emotions along with us.

I felt that it was time to go home and live my life better than I had been doing. I was grateful to know that no one . . . no one knew that I was here this day doing what I was doing and why I was doing it. People deal with pain and grief in some very unusual ways I guess. I have to always do things my own way, and if this helped me, then that is what I needed to do.

I stood up and brushed the dirt from my jeans. I felt much better now. I ran my hand over the polished granite one last time. I chuckled as it occurred to me that I spend way too much time talking to dead people. I think it's something which I became aware of at a very early age and it seemed quite natural to me. I never believed that the connection to a loved one was gone simply because they had died. I believed they were still quite aware of us and they share in our joys and sorrows as we journey through life.

I believed that those who have passed were waiting patiently for us on the other side, waiting for us to complete our tasks and learn our lessons before we are reunited with them again. I once read . . . "Our family chain is broken, nothing seems the same. But as God calls us one by one, the links shall join again.'' I'll see you again someday Anne, and we will be nicer to each other. I promise. In the name of the Father, the Son and the Holy Spirit, Amen. Oh, by the way, did you really stick out your foot from the great beyond and trip Eleanor???

# XXXII
## Welcome to My World

Sweet, sweet acceptance . . . I finally got it. The latest book about Alzheimer's Disease I am now reading said to think about all of the changes we had experienced over time, all the challenges we took on and the problems we were able to solve. It said to congratulate ourselves for being flexible, caring and hard working. It told me to remember that no one can make the disease go away. I'm a very slow learner and quite stubborn, but nonetheless, I finally got it.

Maybe it was the power of prayer. I am sure that it helped me in very subtle ways which I didn't recognize along the way, but I feel that prayer helped me find my own way, and helped me to find my spirit again. For me, it was as if I had woken up one morning and everything was different. I had made it through to the other end of this long internal struggle. I still could not bring myself to congratulate myself for my successes as the book instructed me to do, but I took a deep breath instead and it felt good. I felt good.

It wasn't any one particular incident which caused this sudden change about the way I was looking at life. It was more like years of struggling with each incident, both large and small had finally just brought me to this point of understanding. It wasn't even experiencing the reality of my own jeopardized mortality which woke me up. It wasn't the failures along the way and it wasn't the small successes which woke me up. It wasn't fear, anger, exhaustion, sorrow or any small bit of happiness which woke me up. It wasn't even hashing out my grievances with Anne after all of these years. It wasn't words of wisdom from any one particular source. It wasn't any of these things, yet it was all of these things.

I had been in trouble for seven years. I hadn't realized it at first. What I realize now is that I needed to stop this downward self-destructive direction which I was taking. I needed to change my focus, my direction and get going again. I had a life to lead. That was my job. Each of these life's experiences was meant for a reason. Things in life were going to happen just as they should. Regardless of how much I was anguishing over each event, things were going to continue to happen.

I needed to stop and just let go of the anguish. First, I needed to let it all out. It was going to come out eventually one way or the other. I was holding back all of the things I needed to say out loud and once I did, I could just let it go. Good heavens . . . there are certain things in life that were beyond my control. That thought was a bit unnerving. I wanted my life back more than anything in the world. I simply needed to accept the things I could not change and accept Dad's world for what it was, and on his terms. It was the only way to free myself from this new loop I found myself caught up in.

I checked myself all over and to my surprise, I was still in one piece. There was something very calming about accepting defeat this time. It didn't mean I had failed. In fact, it wasn't really defeat at all. It was success. It was heavily camouflaged success, but nonetheless, it was success because we had done our best. I had done my best. Accepting Dad's struggle for what it was didn't at all mean that I stopped loving him. In fact, I loved him all the more for teaching me just a few more of life's precious valuable lessons, in his own very special way. If I had not been chosen to accompany Walter on his journey, I never would have grown through all of these experiences. My life never would have been touched by all of those wonderful people I had met along the way. I never would have appreciated the things I do have to the degree which I do now.

My new revelation has finally put things into perspective. Walter is continuing along his path in life. He is doing nothing different than he was at the beginning of this long journey. He is progressing gently and quietly through each stage as if everything were in control, untouched and as it should be. The only difference is a new perspective from his back seat driver. I took this job very seriously. I viewed Promise Number Three as the most important mission of my life. Nothing can change what had happened along the journey, and I am not going to create another loop for myself. I am not going to relive the events over and over again, struggling to change the ending. I don't want to change the ending. It is as it should be. The difference is me and my understanding of how I have grown since the journey began. The journey itself changed me in so many ways.

I reflected on how I spiraled out of control so many times, trying to function and finding my own way in a frustrated panicked frenzy. I wanted to fix things. I was always in search of normalcy. I was always afraid of letting Walter down. I was afraid of letting Anne down. I didn't want to fail. I was looking for answers which would never be found. The journey reminded me of something I had read about the stages you go through when dealing with the death of a loved one.

All of the stages rang true. There was shock, fear, grief, denial, mourning and finally acceptance. I experienced all of these things. Mourning is difficult when the one you love is gone yet still alive. There is no closure. Acceptance is such a great thing. Years later, it seems simple. It was all really about one thing. Life was going on in the way it was supposed to whether I liked it or not. I had done my best and at the end of each day, that was all that really mattered.

I had a dream about my own Dad that night. I dreamt that I drove to his house and the road, yard and the driveway was filled with cars I didn't recognize. I slowly made my way into the house walking past strangers who didn't even seem to notice I was there. The rooms were filled with murmuring guests, everyone speaking so softly that I couldn't understand anyone. I couldn't find my Dad. He was not there. Who were all of these people? What were they doing there? Why were they all dressed up? Why is it that I don't know anyone? Why is it that when I talk to them, they are not seeing or acknowledging me? I woke up. It was 2:33 A.M. and I was looking at the ceiling fan again. One didn't have to be a genius to figure out that I was subconsciously preparing myself for the day he decides to leave us. I thought that I had better go and see him that night after work.

The dream bothered me all day long. I think it was because it was so vivid. I could picture it clearly, right down to the makes and models of the cars I didn't recognize in the yard. I had detailed recollections of the clothes that the total strangers were wearing. Everything was vividly clear except for what they were saying, just soft murmurs were all I could hear. Usually memories of my dreams stayed with me for only a minute or two after I woke, but this one was different.

Something was wrong. That night after work I made my way down the country road toward his house. I was relieved to see that there were no cars on the road, in his yard or driveway. I let out a little sigh of relief. Dreams can be funny at times. I once again was making something out of nothing.

I found my Dad sitting on the couch, watching the news as usual. I let out a second sigh of relief. I chuckled to myself and I shook my head. The perfect epitaph for my stone popped into my head . . . "Died a Thousand Deaths . . . Buried only Once." The perfect description of someone in constant worry and panic mode. How about this one instead . . . "Idiot Girl." There must be a medical term for someone always waiting in fear, on the brink and waiting for the sky to fall down. There must be a "something-or-other . . . noia or phobia" with my name on it. I'll have to remind myself to look that up someday when I have time. I never lived like that when I was younger and I need to stop. My Dad stood up to give me my customary kiss in the middle of my forehead.

We sat down and I asked my Dad what was new. Within a few minutes time, he told me the exact same story three times. He told me that his sister Mary had called him from Florida. They had a long conversation. I asked what they had talked about and he would think for a minute and tell me he couldn't remember. A minute or two later, he would again announce that his sister Mary had called him from Florida . . . talked for a long time . . . couldn't remember what was said . . . and so it went. I listened. When he was all done telling me what he needed to say, I kissed him goodbye. On my short drive home, I wondered if I had any unresolved issues with my Dad. Jeeze . . . after almost fifty years you'd think I might have a little list going on there. I did not. I honestly did not and the awareness of that thought made me feel incredibly good.

Walter taught me a couple of things here which might be useful. I am not wasting my time on shock, denial, fear, anger, panic or any steps in between. I am not going through the grueling bar-lowering ritual. I am skipping all of that and am going right to acceptance. First of all, I understand

201

that older people sometimes or should I say often repeat themselves. Everyone knows that. It's probably not a good thing that his repetitive stories follow in immediate identical sequence three times in a row like that but let's face it, I shall never be an expert on tangled ganglion fibers and the human brain. Second of all, Aunt Mary lives in Massachusetts, not Florida and I don't think she has ever even visited Florida. Since there is little or no chance of me bribing her to move south, just so Dad's story can be correct, I must accept the extent of his confusion and condition without all of the emotional destruction to myself.

Do you see what is going on here? Do you see how great I am getting at this? No falling apart, no panicked frenzy. No "loops" in sight. No more big giant holes torn in my tapestry. Walter had a good student. I drove home and impressed David with the details of what had happened and how well I had handled myself. This was a sad thing which was now happening to my Dad, but I would be a better daughter to him by keeping my head on straight. After some time, I noticed that David was studying me quietly with a tiny smile on his lips. My monologue was broken mid-stream as I stopped to ask him why he was looking at me that way. His smile got bigger as he gently patted my arm. "Do you realize that you have just told me that same story, start to finish, three times in a row?"

I think about Walter, but I do not think about Walter all of the time as I once did, and not in the same way. It seemed as though I wasn't in the thick of it emotionally anymore. It was more like I was just watching and caring from a distance. I began to truly appreciate the things I had learned from Walter and his struggle, and I was sure that Walter had gently changed the lives all of the people who loved him and even strangers whose lives he had touched.

He was truly amazing in his own quiet way. Walter had created a beautiful tapestry with his life. Mine on the other hand, could still use some work. As things began to come back into perspective for me, I could almost feel the tattered and bunched fabric relaxing and the twisted mess of my knots unraveling. I am going to need to do a little repair work. Although the tell-tale signs of damage will always remain, this is one piece of fabric that can be repaired. In fact, the little flaws left behind will give it some character.

I thought I might call an old friend who I had pushed away a long time ago. I don't know. They wouldn't know me any more, but maybe I can try. I thought I might challenge myself a bit too. I think I might raise my own bar, just this once. I could take on a challenge and start writing again. They say you should write about what you know. Albert Einstein once said, "There is no knowledge without experience." I might just have one or two interesting experiences in my life which I could write about. Taking on a challenge is sometimes a little scary, especially for me. If you don't take a chance, you can avoid a lot of disappointments and failures by playing it safe instead, but you are also cheating yourself out of an occasional success. I think I will go for it.

I thought about the friends I once had again. I missed friendship. I had become cynical almost overnight it seemed. Maybe it was anger or resentment which fueled the fire. It seemed to me that I had been dealt a really crappy hand somewhere down the road and I felt that I didn't deserve it. I found it hard to fit in with those whose lives appeared to be going along fine. I would listen in silence as others would complain about meaningless obstacles affecting their world. I remembered wanting to leave the room shrieking once when a friend's day was completely ruined because they had broken a fingernail. How could I possibly confide my innermost feelings of being lost with someone like that?

I distanced myself because I had decided that true friends were far and few between. I became very conscious of those who I saw as judgmental "fair-weather friends." Sadly, the term could have also been "fair-weather family." It was a term I used to describe people who only seemed to come around when times were good, fleeing at the first sign of sadness or trouble. People who seemed to appear only when they needed something. I alienated some very great well-meaning people in the process.

One day I opened the paper to discover that the elderly father of one of my friends from long ago had died after being ill in a nursing home for over a year. I felt so selfish and ashamed for feeling like I was the only person in the world going through life-changing hardships. I wanted to make things right and apologize to her, and to make amends for judging others so harshly.

It turned out that my old friend had never stopped caring about me, and frequently had stopped to ask David how I was holding up over the years. I was the one who was that "fair-weather friend" after all. I had somewhere down the road, convinced myself that no one would care about this new different person I had become. I felt that since that old happy free-spirited smiling person I once was had gone, they would not care to know the person I had become. I realized that I was wrong, that there were many good people that did care. I never had given them a chance, and that I was the one, not them, who hastily ditched friendship at the first sign of trouble.

I still had a watchful eye out for those who appeared only when they needed something, usually something self-serving or trivial in my opinion as I really hated that kind of thing, but I really needed to examine my own judgmental behavior of late, or I had a feeling I will never let anyone become close to me again. That would be a real shame. By the way, who hasn't let out a spew of frustration over breaking a nail? It didn't mean that one small incident was a reflection of their character, it only meant that they were human. Most likely they were just having a bad day, or maybe even more serious troubles of their own. Maybe I should have taken a moment to listen.

I would be very lucky indeed to find just one friend after how I have behaved. There was something rather disturbing, even to me, that my only friend during this struggle was Maggie. Maggie . . . a woman I had never met. She was a woman of conviction and a faithful daughter. A hardworking care giver with all the right intentions. As my story began, I had really only read her obituary in the paper when I first felt a connection with her. Yes, Maggie would have understood and yes, her story was so shockingly sad and painfully real to me. But sadly, I became convinced that no one else could ever really understand how I felt or what I was going through unless they had walked in my shoes. I think a friend would have understood if I had just given them a chance. This is something I really hope I can change.

Today was an exciting day which began with an interesting phone call. It seems that there exists a Granite Guild Association in Barre, VT. This is the place where granite is cut from the huge quarries and is used for many purposes, much of which is used in the production of memorial stones. The guild consists of officers, trustees, staff and an advisory board which put together a publication. The publication consists of articles, photographs of interesting works done and various advertisements relating to the trade. Well, it seems that they chose a large photograph of my beautifully carved Celtic Cross stone to grace the cover of their latest addition.

I shook my head and laughed out loud. Only in America! I gave the guild office my address and several days later, a box arrived with twenty or so copies of the publication. Sure enough, the cover was graced with a beautiful large color photograph of my stone, complete with my name, my family's village name in Ireland and my humorous epitaph all in Gaelic and carved Celtic knots. The stone was beautiful, a work of art. It was really something and I was strangely amused. One of my goals in life was to have something I wrote published, and there it was! My humorous epitaph, my famous last words of all things! My Dad was going to laugh for an hour and my Irish cousins would be so proud. He did, they were . . . and they all wanted copies.

I must be special. I am the only person I have ever known who had such interesting and amusing things like this happen to them in their life. Okay, so what does this rather bizarre bit of amusement mean? I can't help but think that someone upstairs is displaying his sense of humor again, or maybe he is reminding me to keep mine as well. My grave stone prominently displayed on the cover of a nationwide publication? How funny is that? And now I can honestly tell people that I have been a Cover Girl! Secretly, I was very proud of my creation and most thrilled to see it in glossy color print. I shall try to not let all of the fame change me much.

Maybe, just maybe, my recent not so subtle sign from above was to remind me of who I was. I hoped it wasn't a reminder of my pending mortality. I choose to think of it more as a humorous postcard from God, if you will. I decided to pick up where I left off with my genealogy project. To me, it's like reuniting with long lost friends. I ordered some new microfiche from County Cork and County Kerry. They are supposed to contain some newly discovered old church records. There are family members waiting to be found. I'm in heaven! I dusted off my old microfiche reader and reorganized my little office here at home.

Something tells me I still have a few exciting adventures just waiting for me down the road. I feel as though the key to my new adventure might just be found in that envelope containing the microfiche. That envelope is Par-Avion-ing its way to me right this very moment. I'll bet there are several more beautiful Celtic Crosses to be discovered somewhere along that road too. Life is good.

I've been spending some time in my perennial garden. I have been quite neglectful these past few years. It has really fallen to wreck and ruin. I can just envision the beautiful whimsical English garden I had once been so proud of. My roses are a mess. I bought three new stone pillars which will look lovely once strategically placed in my new and improved garden. I can picture them supporting some lovely old urns with beautiful pink flowers cascading over their rims. I'll need some cobblestones too, and tons of mulch. I'm thinking it could use a small stone bench. The lovely little brook is still gently rippling as it winds its way behind the garden. Its banks are overgrown though. I love the sound of that brook. It has been a long time since I really stopped to listen to it.

I poked around through the tall weeds in search of my lavender plants. They look droopy and tired, but they are still alive. They just need a little care. I bent down and rubbed their dry leaves thought my fingers. The aroma of lavender was wonderful. It was like I was smelling it for the first time. It reminded me of Dad, seeing the sunset and watching in wonderment as if he was seeing it for the first time. This restoration project is going to require a lot of work, but I'm up to the challenge. This is something I can fix. Now, if I could just find my tools. Where did I put my tools? My eyes wandered over to our old compost pile at the end of our property. No, I'm not going over there. It will just have to remain one of life's great mysteries.

I looked up from my garden at our beautiful house. I don't think I ever realized just how pretty it was. It was ours, bought and paid for. We had saved every penny for fifteen years just for the down payment. I loved that house and we spent the first several years in our new home devoting every free moment and every last dollar to fixing it up. There had been some really tough times, and a few especially difficult times when I worried about scraping up the mortgage payment. We always pulled through. All of our hard work, and it's finally paid off. It is time that I appreciated the simple blessings, starting with the things that were right here, right in my own backyard.

Years ago, when I was all of eighteen and most full of self-proclaimed wisdom, I had this driving urge to leave the little town I grew up in to see the world. I could not find one little piece of ingratiating goodness in the quiet backwoods and country small town way of life. I was bursting to escape, find adventures, meet different people, visit faraway places and experience life in places that surely had to be better and much more exciting than where I had come from. Well, I did all of those things and years later I wanted a home of my own. I had searched far and wide, only to find that the most beautiful place on earth was the little town I had fled from. My home is less than three miles from the house I grew up in. Funny . . . isn't it?

It had been my safe-haven for these past seven years. It was set far back in the woods, not visible from the road. The little brook crossed under the windy driveway. The house was hidden by the dense trees from other neighbors. It was on a very quiet dead-end street. It became a place where I could escape from the outside world. I couldn't see out and no one could see in. For years, I felt that it was my own little piece of "Brigadoon." As any movie buff remembers, the breathtaking beauty of Brigadoon materializes from the Scottish mist only one day every hundred years in the movies. The eighteenth century residents were safe, happy, protected and sheltered from the outside world as long as they never left the village. It was a nice story.

Brigadoon may have seemed like the perfect place to be, but you woke up to discover that all of your friends and family, all the people and things you cared about outside of the mystical ethereal village had vanished while you were sleeping. When the sun rose through the mist the following morning in Brigadoon, a hundred years had really passed in the outside world. All of their problems just vanished like a long ago memory. It was not really so perfect after all. Of course in the movie, it was love that brought an outsider in to live out his life in sheltered happiness.

For me, happiness was to be found only when I could muster enough courage to cross over the bridge into the real world where I could start living life again. I had become what could be described as an emotional "shut-in," still functioning, but almost as if I were two different people. I was who I wanted everyone else to see me as, and I was who I really was within the sheltered walls of my home.

I looked up at the house again. It looked a little neglected, a little faded and in need of some repair. Some of the cedar clapboards needed replacing. There was some water damage to the moldings around the front door. I was bothered as I thought about the other unfinished projects. The upstairs bathroom was never quite finished either. We had started taping the seams of the bare sheet rock and it was almost done, but for some reason, seven years ago we had just stopped. Life just seemed to have stopped. It stayed that way, untouched for years. That was not like me. I always saw things through until the end. I was never satisfied to leave details undone. A little joint compound, a little sanding, a little paint and a little paper was all that was needed. A trip or two to Home Depot is all it will take to finish it. This was something I could fix.

I special ordered some new wallpaper and matching border for one of the bedrooms. It was coming from England and it was beautiful, rich and full of color. It had a very pleasing Victorian look about it. I was never really happy with the way those plain white painted walls looked for years. It is time for a fresh new look and I should be able to put it all up in one weekend if I roll up my sleeves and get going. This was something I could fix. I walked around to the back yard. I hadn't noticed until now how all of the small shrubbery I had lovingly planted years ago on the bare hillside had now grown and had filled in nicely. I was glad that nature had taken care of itself, as I had been somewhere else. I knocked the dirt off of my shoes and went inside. My cat, Patrick, gave me his trademark disinterested yawn and went and sat by his empty food dish. Isn't it nice to know that some things never change?

I pulled back the curtains and opened all of the windows. The sun shone though and lovely shadows danced across the walls. Hmmmm . . . I noticed a couple of cobwebs in the far corners of the window frames that seemed to come to life with the fresh cool breeze passing through. I wonder how long those had been there? Probably as long as that dust bunny, which had now made its home in the neglected far corner of the room. Maybe I could just name it "Fluffy" and look the other way. What is happening here?? The next thing you know, I will be saying it's okay to eat crackers in bed! The new me is not going to sweat the small stuff anymore and I am going to just sit back and enjoy life . . . no . . . no I'm not . . . some old habits die hard and "Fluffy" will have to go. This will be the first item on my list of to-do's.

Cleaning always cheers me up. I am in control of the vacuum cleaner if nothing else. I like things tidy and in order. I rummaged through closets and drawers looking for things which were no longer important and could be discarded. I came across my old high school yearbook which had been buried for almost thirty years now. It seemed like only yesterday, and I chuckled as I flipped through the pages. I was sporting some really interesting clothes and hairdos back then. I felt my smile begin to fade as I realized that some of my classmates were no longer with us. I began to read some of the sentiments scrawled in pen between the pages, written to me by friends during the frenzy of graduation week. There were the usual recounts of fun and frolic, and many well-wishings as I was soon to embark on my exciting adventures in the Navy.

There were other things written as well. Many references to my spirit and zest for life. They all seemed to say the same thing. One girl wrote . . . "Janet! . . . why is it that an exclamation point always follows your name!" It seems as though I was always able to bring excitement and laughter into almost any situation. I had a take-charge way, almost a stampeding approach to life in general, and I just couldn't wait to get out there and do something important. I just knew I would be a success at whichever path I chose. Yep . . . I was marked for success. It had to be. After all, there it was, written in black and white between all of these pages. All of these people saw it too. Hmmm . . . a lot of time has passed. I'm glad those people will never know I was lost in the woods.

One would think by now that I would have it all figured out, but there isn't a day that goes by that I haven't learned something new . . . truly. In a way, that's kind of nice. For all of the reading I have been doing, you would think that I would have some kind of a profound understanding of

Alzheimer's Disease by now but I do not. Nonetheless, I persevere. Today I learned that studies have shown that Omega 3's may be important. They stated that research in Iceland, where a diet rich in cold water fish, and fish oil consumption may somehow have direct benefits with assorted health issues, and they mentioned a connection to aging and Alzheimer's. If I can remember, tomorrow I will go online and order some.

My boss enlightened me with interesting international news today as well. It seems that somewhere over in Ireland or England, he couldn't quite remember, they have come up with an interesting study. It's a pilot program of sorts and quite ingenious if you ask me. They have experimentally located pubs in several of the nursing homes. Morale has improved considerably as now the lonely and deserted halls echo with laughter and cheer. Suddenly visitors are showing up by the busload to visit the once forgotten. A win-win situation for all. How advanced they are across the ocean! How simple . . . just make an enjoyable environment, kind of a "if you build it . . . they will come" idea. I was amused, and yet a little envious that I wasn't the one to come up with that idea myself.

I could picture myself tipping a pint or two with the rest of the forlorn family members as we sorted out all of life's trials and tribulations. No . . . this journey is a long one. A very long one and alcohol is a depressant. Society does not need a sudden surge of alcoholics emerging as a new side effect from this ever growing population of Alzheimer's families. There are already so many ups and downs, that sometimes it becomes hard to distinguish which is which.

In reflection, how easily all of those emotionally charged moments rolled into minutes, then hours, then days, weeks, months and now years. This passage of time has now marked another year. This has been one long exhaustive journey for all of us, and we are still not there. We have accepted the reality that Walter may continue on for many more years in his unknown and misunderstood world. There are now no more emotionally charged moments. It seems all quite peaceful, in fact. We have all changed. Some of us more than others.

We went to visit Walter again, and now I find myself wondering each time if it will be our last visit. The occasion at the facility this time was a fall festival. We arrived to the familiar sounds of Glenn Miller, and the place smelled like baked chicken, apple crisp and cider. We were in Dad's room and David was applying zinc cream to Walter's legs and arms. They seemed to be getting worse. We had a visitor. He was a frail old bent-over type of quiet man who just shuffled in to watch. He studied David for a long time. He watched him carefully as David attended to Walter's wounds. Then he said "That man really knows what he is doing."

Walter looked confused. "What man?" he asked, "I don't see a man."

"David," I said, "he's talking about David."

"Well . . . who is David?" he asked.

In walked another visitor. She was a small frail woman and she wore a visibly upset face. She appeared to be in her early eighties. "What's wrong?" I asked. Through teary eyes she gazed at me. She then blurted out, "My name is Alice. I live at 14 Arch Street and I need to go home." She sobbed as she told me she didn't have any money, but asked if could I please take her back home. She told me "they" just dumped her here and she didn't know what to do. She told me again, "My name is Alice. I live at 14 Arch Street and I need to go home." I took her by the hand and told her that everything was going to be alright. I told her I would help her find her room. She became irritated with me. This place

213

was not her home. How many times did she have to tell me . . . Her name was Alice. She lived at 14 Arch Street, and she needed to go home. This was not her home.

The sad part about this story is that Alice, like Walter, still knew too much when she was brought here. Her transition was going to be long and painful for her. I sadly took her by the hand and made our way around the four sections of the facility looking for a nurse, an aide, or anybody who could help me to help Alice find her way back to her room. I thought I could go with her and have a little look at the shadow box. I could try to make her feel better by striking up a conversation using some clue I gathered from her photos. I could do this, I could do that . . . no, I can't. Finally I found an aide who gathered up Alice and directed her to her room. I turned to walk away, her voice still ringing in my head, "My name is Alice. I live at 14 Arch Street and I need to go home . . . "

I walked back down the hall making my way toward the music and the festivities. David and Walter had to be around there somewhere. I saw Patrick bee-bopping along. He flashed me a big giant smile and told me he was looking for his "sleeve holder." This was his pet name for Katie as she held his sleeve when they walked together. I smiled as I watched his almost animated face. Patrick always had this special way about him. He was really something. Who ever called their wife their "sleeve holder" anyway? Only my friend Patrick.

I darted out of the path of Tilly and her walker. I learned a long time ago that when you hear that thing coming, it's best to move swiftly. Tilly was headed toward the music. That meant that David was probably on the lookout for her, nervously hiding in some closet or at least cowering in a shadow. Tilly slowed down a little when she saw me. I noticed the buttons on her sweater were still not matching up right, her hair was a frightful mess and her Halloween pin was on upside down. I thought for a minute before I asked. I already knew the answer but I asked anyway. "Tilly . . . can I help you fix your pin?"

She replied, "Oh no dear . . . I already fixed it myself." With that, she whizzed down the hall like her little wheels were on fire. Who else could be so independently sure of herself? Only my friend Tilly.

Walter's pace had really slowed to a crawl but I found him still smiling and keeping up with the music on the dance floor. One of the nurses was dancing with him. I made my way toward a sitting area where I found David. We both just sat and watched Walter as he smiled and danced. I could tell that David felt a little sad when Dad did not acknowledge him by his name. The song was over and the nurse was guiding Walter back toward us. I could hear her saying "Walter, why don't you dance with your daughter?" He was looking all over the place for this would-be daughter. By now I was right in front of him, standing up, calling out his name and waving my arms. He wasn't seeing me. She was still saying to him "Your daughter, Walter, she's right there."

Walter's eyes slowly searched the room. His face seemed expressionless. I still found myself wishing I could understand what his world must have looked like to him. I wondered if it was like being in a cloudy dream, where you follow along with the unclear and confusing story. You may sometimes understand bits of it, but mostly you watch as the rest of it passes before your eyes with a confused blur. As with a lot of dreams which I can recall, you know it doesn't make sense but you agreeably go along with it anyway.

Walter looked down at a ninety-year-old woman sitting in a chair. He asked the nurse, "Is this my daughter?" I sat back down next to David and flashed him a little smile and rolled my eyes. I was okay with it. Still, Walter could have at least had the decency to confuse me with some younger, stunningly beautiful type of female in the room, but no, he confused me with the ninety-year-old white-haired woman who was staring blankly into space—and I'm pretty sure she was drooling. Still, you've got to love him.

Dad sat down to eat but he seemed to struggle with the utensils. I noticed lately that he studies them, not sure anymore as to how they work. He studies his food as well like he is wondering what it is all about. Eventually he gets the idea on feeding himself, maybe from watching others, I don't know. From time to time, I still find myself trying to come to reason with Dad's view of the world. I think of my own pleasant incidences or events, for example when I have heard from a long lost relative, or have spoken to someone who has impacted my life in some positive way. Their contact remains with me as a warm memory for days, weeks, months or longer. I am conscious of how many times I revisit those warm moments.

I am grateful for the way the mind allows us to just retrieve certain special moments and re-live the feelings which go along with these memories. It's as though I can reach into my well organized memory filing cabinet and pull out what I need. It is so amazing how the memory works. That is how I see it from my world. It really bugs me that I can't see what Walter is seeing. I have always wanted so badly to understand. He doesn't know us but he seems to respond to us anyway. Somewhere in his mind, we must still be im- printed as a good or caring memory. We seem to connect with him during our visits on some level. He seems able to retrieve this imprinted feeling for the moment only. When we get up to leave, the imprint seems to lift up and blow away.

I often wonder if his world is empty or void of thought, or is it a tornado of whirling bits of tangled information. I wonder if his thoughts are very quiet, or if they are loud. One will never know if our visits have meaning. I think they do, if only for a moment. Maybe we are making his world a little better in some small way. In my heart, I know we are doing the right thing. It's not important to understand how or why this time.

I had a dream that night. You know, I really must buy a book on the subject as I am exhausted trying to decipher the deep hidden meanings of all of this stuff I am constantly hashing out each night in my sleep. In this nocturnal adventure, it seems I was at a deserted carnival. There was no one else in sight. That didn't seem to bother me at all, and I climbed onto this ride that spins around and around in a circle. On the seat were a pair of 3–D cardboard glasses, the kind they used to have in the old movie theaters I think. Anyway, I put the glasses on and seemed quite excited for the ride to begin.

Music began and the ride started. Around and around I went, thinking how amazing and clear the world looked through three dimensional glasses. I remember enjoying myself until the music began to fade. At first faintly, I could make out a voice replacing the music. It was a woman's voice repeating over and over again ''My name is Alice . . . I want to go home . . . '' The voice was getting louder and angrier. I couldn't see her and the ride wouldn't stop. I began spinning faster and faster and I was beginning to panic. It was at that point that I abruptly woke up. It was 1:53 A.M. and I am wide awake and sweaty. I can hear the sound of my heart beating rapidly in my chest.

I am supposed to be getting better, yet it seems as though each time I cross paths with another lost soul, I become upset on some level and need to come to terms with it. Since I had four hours to kill before I needed to go to work, I decided to think about the dream. The first thing that came to mind was guilt. I walked away from Alice at the facility when she was obviously confused, alone and upset. I could have gotten more involved and I didn't. I didn't want to learn anything about her or her life from her shadow box because it is just too difficult for me. I helped her only to a point and then I turned my back. It was very difficult doing that. It did not feel right.

This disease to me is like no other. It is a silent killer which first erases your mind, your memories of everything important to you in your life. It takes your identity away from you. Then it eventually robs you of physical abilities, slowly and without dignity until you die. Every face in the facility is destined for the same cruel end. My heart breaks for Dad, whom I love. My heart breaks for total strangers who are lost and upset. All of these people made a difference here on earth. Some made significant contributions, some made small contributions. The point is that it mattered . . . it mattered that each one of these individuals was here, and this disease could steal everything but that. With Alice, I tried to protect myself a little bit by keeping a safe distance. I too easily become attached to these residents. A brief encounter is all it would take anyone before they are touched by the reality of what is happening to these people.

Alright, alone at a carnival. I haven't been to a carnival in years, but nonetheless, I think the point was that I was alone. Maybe I chose a carnival because it is a place where families come to have fun. There should be sounds of laughter, happy children and happy faces yet I am, or I chose to be alone. I don't even like rides particularly, but nonetheless I was on one. I chose to get on a ride which goes nowhere, it just spins around and around aimlessly in a big circle. You pass by the same objects again and again until it all becomes a repetitive blur.

I think that it is interesting that 3-D cardboard glasses were waiting for me on my seat. These were not rose-colored glasses, I know this because I checked. I must have really wanted to see the full perspective, a different view, all dimensions, or come to some kind of understanding if you will. I only know I wanted it to stop, I wanted to get off and go home. A very interesting dream indeed and it probably meant little, but I'm thinking someday when I am very old and quite wise, I may understand. For now, I think I'll get ready for work.

The air was getting cooler. The air even smells like fall and the leaves are changing. I can smell a hint of smoke from a far away neighbor's fireplace. I wonder if I still have that pumpkin-colored sweater with the tiny buttons? I think I'll go through the closets and see what I can get rid of. There is something very liberating about letting go of old, meaningless junk. I am looking forward to putting the chrysanthemums and the pumpkins out on the front steps this year. Who knows, I might just have to take a little ride north to that "State Owned" land and swipe myself some nice Bittersweet to put on the mantel. Christmas will be different this year. I can feel it.

I drove past Mom and Dad's old house. Although it was always visible from the road I took every day to and from work, I guess I would subconsciously look the other way. Today I looked at it with interest. The new owners had given it a fresh coat of paint. They had pulled out the old shrubs near the foundation which had been terribly overgrown for years. I smiled as I thought of Mom. She was always asking Walter to remove them but he never would. She would have liked the way it now looked. The new owners also put up quaint shutters. That was one little detail that I had always thought was needed and now, the somewhat neglected Cape Cod-style homestead really seemed to take on a new charm of its own. The new owners cared about the little house and I felt good about that.

David and Raymond are still struggling with the sale of Dad's property. It's now years later and the issue seems still firmly planted at square one. They went to another town zoning meeting last week to try and move things forward. The meeting was adjourned until next month, pending further proposals. The potential buyers backed out after several years of environmental studies. I suppose it will sell, like everything else, in its own good time. They had to meet with the man from the state, something to do with the water testing. I am not worried. I have removed myself from such things. No, I take that back. I am not quite as removed as I proclaim. I still feel the urge to vent about one last issue. Well . . . the last for now anyway.

If my calculations are correct, and with the property sale falling through and at a standstill, Dad will be out of funds in about seven to eight months. This means we must get him to a nursing home as soon as possible, immediately, if not sooner. So it appears to me that this move at this particular time is not specifically medically indicated. We have no desire to pull him from his environment which is solely dedicated to the care of Alzheimer's residents as this is now his home and his environment in which he is comfortable and secure on whatever level that may be. The bottom line is money. As I said when this story began, this part of the bargain did not leave me with warm and fuzzy feelings as indicated by the brochures.

I digress. To live in this facility at all, one needs money, and plenty of it. Rule number one . . . they are private companies of sorts, not considered nursing homes, and not mandated to accept Title 19. You are a resident in good standing as long as you still have cash and as long as your condition does not require extensive special care. Apparently, as one's condition advances, they are required to be moved to a nursing home. Hmmmm . . . I am flashing back to a simpler time when none of this seemed real or important, and certainly not urgent. It's now years later and I am still not getting that warm fuzzy feeling they want you to get when they show their TV commercials of your aging parent skipping through the daisies at their facility. Whether the property was sold or not, Dad would be in this same boat, only the timing would be different.

Now for the Catch-22. Had Dad's property been sold, he would have had sufficient funds, which would have meant he could live in his current facility for six or seven more years, or until his condition required advanced care at a nursing home. The cost to live at this private company facility is currently about $ 70,000 per year. But because the property is not sold, and actual remaining cash can only sustain him for less than a year, it is imperative that we move him to a more expensive facility, a nursing home, at a cost of $ 108,000 per year to establish his residence as a "paying customer" for a period of time before the funds run out and he must apply for Title 19. So the poor man is running out of money and the obvious solution is to move him to a more expensive facility, even if not medically indicated and away from a facility which is solely dedicated to his disease. Have I missed something?

Will someone please explain to me why more expensive nursing homes are required to accept Title 19, yet these Alzheimer's facilities are not? In our area, these Alzheimer's facilities cost less per year than the nursing homes, somewhere in the range of 25% less. Why can't allotted funds directed toward the nursing homes be redirected toward the Alzheimer's facility instead? Can someone out there please figure out a way for these poor residents to remain where they are? After all, aren't they just the silent victims with no choice in their terrible destiny? It's not like they are trying to sneak themselves a free stay at a county club for God's sake.

My loud tirade will not be heard over bureaucratic driveling as I know not of what I speak. I know only of what I feel to be basic when it comes to what is right and what is wrong. With Dad, there was only one thing to be done. David and his brother reluctantly made an appointment with a nursing home in the area to view the facility and prepare for the move. In talking with a lot of people over the past several years, we had heard all kinds of stories, both good and bad about the several nursing homes in the area. We ran into a man we knew with a loved one in a facility close by not long ago. We asked our usual question about if the family was happy with the facility. It has been my experience that family members will be more than willing to dish out the dirt if they are not completely satisfied, and we waited for his vigorous response.

He thought for a good long minute before he answered. He said that it was his opinion that all of the nursing homes in our area, with the exception of a notable problem home which is frequently in the media, all had their good and their bad, all incredibly expensive. He said that he thought the more important issue was the responsibility of Dad's family. He said that it was important that we found a place close enough so that Dad was accessible to friends and family. He quietly and sensitively explained that the most important part of the process, regardless of which place we chose, was letting the staff know that Dad would be visited often, at different hours of the day or night, and that it was clear that we expected to find that he was being cared for properly. In order for us to follow through with that, we needed to be close by.

It was an interesting answer and one which I respected. It wasn't the usual spewing of both really good or really bad about the same places, depending on who you were talking to which left us back in square one. We decided to try to get Dad on the waiting list at a newer facility close by. This nursing home was only eleven years old. It was nice enough, modern and had three floors. I believe men and women were segregated to different floors. The bottom floor seemed to be mostly administrative. The facilities coordinator produced an impressive menu and also an activity list to indicate what was provided for the residents. The rooms were shared, two men to a room, two small closets, one bathroom. One cannot bring their own furniture as they could in Dad's current facility but that is understandable.

The nursing home itself sits poignantly on a hillside overlooking part of the valley. The rooms all have large picture windows and present a panoramic view for any resident interested enough to look out. Ironically, one can stand by any one of the large windows facing north, and see a lovely old country cemetery perched up on a little knoll not far away. This is the place where Mom rests as she waits for Dad to finish his journey. I feel at peace as I know she will be watching over him from a distance, but not all that far.

I am really hoping this will work for both Dad and the other gentleman, whoever he might be. This facility is not just for Alzheimer's, it is for everyone. That means Dad will not know which stuff is his, meaning which bed, which clothes, which belongings which may complicate things for the roommate. Dad also continues with the non-trainable bathroom habits. I just don't want anyone to be angry with Dad for the way he is now. I also don't want some other poor little old man to be miserable having to live with Dad. This place is to be Dad's last home. I cry when I think about that and I cry when I think of what we have all been through I guess we have no other choice now but to write Dad's name on the waiting list.

As Walter's move grows nearer, I am starting to have frequent pangs of sadness, especially when I am watching him silently, and from a distance. He has no idea about this change and I am glad for that. Soon Dad will begin the final stretch of his journey. He is about to embark on the last stage of his life's event. It is almost time to take his faded shadow box down from the wall. Maybe it will end up in a drawer or on a closet shelf.

Maybe we can kind of put this issue away for the time being as it seems that it is time again for the Annual Christmas Party over at Dad's facility. Does everyone have so much sadness during the holidays or is it just me? We continue to jolly it up for everyone concerned but I am hoping it just passes quickly and without incident. As expected, Dad didn't know David, although he went willingly enough when David took him to his doctor's appointment earlier that day and returned for a second visit after buying Dad some new pants that afternoon. It was David's third visit today and he was tired and very quiet. I guess I can put a smile on my face and a festive knitted sweater, sporting a smiling reindeer on Dad and we can just pretend that this is fun.

We can also pretend that his legs aren't swollen and covered with sores. The staff is again not putting his prescription cream and special hose on his legs but perhaps it is not appropriate to have a melt-down on this particular holiday occasion. I shall pretend that his room doesn't smell bad just for fun, and it won't bother me too awfully much that some of Dad's belonging are missing again. I'm not sure just whose clothes are hanging here in Dad's closet. They belong to some other person, but what the heck, it's Christmas after all. Jingle bells. Peace on earth. All is calm . . . all is bright. No reaming of the aides until after New Year's—and that's a damn shame. That always cheers me up.

We paused for a moment just outside of Dad's room as we always do and looked into the shadow box. I don't know why I continue to do that, but I keep on hoping for him to have any small sign of recognition of the now faded photos. He recognizes nothing and seems to struggle with focusing on the box itself, as if he is not seeing it at all. I took him by the hand and we slowly walked toward the festivities. Christmas Music was coming from the community room. They hire entertainers, some of which were really great at previous events. Tonight could be fun. I spoke too soon. I was startled by the sight of a 300-pound man in an elf costume, his tights several sizes too small, singing and puffing out "Rudolph the Red Nose Reindeer" on the tuba. Nothing screams out Merry Christmas like the sight of that.

Did anyone hear my huge loud groan of disappointment? I needed a diversion. Here is what I found to be very interesting instead. Dad and other residents had no real recognition of their surroundings or even their families yet they could sing all of the words to the Christmas Carols. Can you see how I distracted myself from the vision of scary elf man by focusing on something which could be more meaningful? I calculated that Dad had no memories of his son. Those memories only went back fifty-three years, but Christmas Carols were a part of his life for seventy-eight years. Those memories must have been so deeply engraved that he was able to somehow retrieve them.

As I looked around the room, I could see the same with others as well as lips moved with the music. Elf man was on a break. That was good, exhausted no doubt after his "interesting" and most theatrical rendition of "The Twelve Days of Christmas." I took Dad gently by the hand and led him to the dance floor. It was a slow song and I held him tight. As the band played, Dad sang every word to "White Christmas" into my ear with perfection as we danced. When the song was finished, he thanked me and he called me "honey." Dad never once in all of these years, ever called me that. In fact, I don't recall him calling anyone "honey." Before we left that night, David punched another hole in Dad's belt. Dad was losing weight. Still, these grueling holidays were becoming a little bit easier to get through for all of us, I think.

I once wondered what Dr. Phil would have said to me if he had found me in the cemetery that day hashing it all out with Anne. I amused myself as I wondered if he would have told me I was doing a spectacular job, like everyone else had been telling me. No . . . he would have easily spotted the shallow façade. One can not fool Dr. Phil. I am thinking he would have instead told me to seek immediate help, using words like "atychiphobia" to describe my fear of failure. Maybe he would point out the severity of my "atelophobia" or "ataxophobia" to describe my fear of imperfection, fear of disorder and untidiness.

No . . . he would have gone directly to "dementophobia" . . . my fear of insanity! And that would be just the beginning. Yep, he would be having a field day here. Perhaps he might have deduced that all factors indicated that I was potty-trained too early. Surely that would explain things. I would have had to tell him that he was a smart man, but he didn't know everything. I was going to find my own way out. I would have had to tell him that all the books in the world could not have begun to touch upon the knowledge and healing given as a special gift to me by a man in the final stage of Alzheimer's Disease.

# XXXIII
## "Life's List"

I pulled out my "Life's List" once more—one more of those old habits which die hard. After all, I still must be organized. This was my road map. It's time to reevaluate what is really important. Hmmmm . . . let's see. Number one on my list: "Live to be a hundred . . . with one extra year to repent." That still sounds pretty good to me. That one stays. Maybe I'll take that cooking class after all. Ha! That's never going to happen. It's best to let that one go. I have learned to accept my limitations. Remember, letting go is sometimes a good thing. I suppose it's not really important that I learn to sky dive either. I guess I should scratch that one off the list too.

Here's one I would love to do, "Take Dad on a Hot Air Balloon Ride." I had meant my own Dad, not Walter. Taking Walter would have been out of the question at this point, although he would have enjoyed it years ago. The balloon launch field was only a few miles away, and I would often see the beautiful balloons drifting silently overhead as I drove to work in the morning. My Dad would love that. We had experienced some pretty interesting adventures together since I was a little girl, and this was something I always wanted to do with him. I guess we will have to wait to see what the doctors have to say about it after his next appointment. This one will be up to God, and I think I will keep it on the list.

"Places to Visit" . . . very interesting. This one has a sublist which is very long. I read the location of each exciting place on the list. I could remember the reason for writing down each place I had listed, even if I had written them down years ago. I think I'll keep them all on the list for now. "Learn Gaelic." This is do-able. I'm not too sure how many riveting conversations I would be having when I was through, but what the heck. It may come in handy someday. "Celebrate St. Patrick's Day on the Streets of Killarney" . . . I will do this someday . . . mark my words! "Restore or Purchase a 50's Classic Car" . . . I can only hope that the boot is large enough to transport my walker, as I could be very old by the time I make this one happen, but . . I think I'll leave it on the list anyway, just for fun.

"Cut Back on Swearing"—that's going to be a damned hard one. It's probably best that I don't push myself too hard with all of these goals. Maybe I can just ease into a few of them gently. "Learn Sign Language" . . . I wonder what prompted me to write that? I can't really remember, but if the opportunity ever presents itself, I'll know it was meant to be. "Go on a Long Distance Train Adventure" . . . still good, "Fly to London to Wave at the Queen" . . . an interesting priority I once had, yet no longer important. "Take a Course in Photography" Hmmmm . . . now this one is a keeper. "Learn to Sing" . . . nope, out of the question. "Dance like Michael Flatley, that Celtic Tiger in Riverdance with his Feet of Flames." Who wrote this list anyway? I think I shall lower my own bar on this one. I'm thinking that I shall place my dancing shoes next to Tilly's as we are surely both in the same league.

"Sleep in a Haunted Castle," "Get Tickets to a NASCAR Race," "Grow a Rose Garden," "Kiss the Blarney Stone," "Get Cable TV Before I Die." Ha! I already did those things, just forgot to cross them off the list. "Get a Shamrock Tattoo on My Ass" . . . must have written down that one after a wild drunken night at a family reunion years ago. This one is still up in the air apparently, as I can't seem to make my pen draw a line thought it. "Spend a Day on Ellis Island" . . . good one. "Know My Neighbors" . . . now there is an interesting one. We had always exchanged pleasantries, but for years now we have pretty much kept to ourselves. "Become a Bone Marrow Donor Match" . . . that one is a big one and is really up to God.

"Don't Sweat the Small Stuff" . . . "Discover a Friend" . . . "Find the Joy in Christmas Again" . . . "Be Kinder To Old People" . . . "Help Someone in Trouble" . . . "Stay Happy" . . . "Go Back to Church." Hmmmm . . . It was interesting that I had written that some time ago. I never would have described myself as a religious person and rarely made an appearance in church. One would see my face there for weddings and funerals only. Yet it seemed as I was working my way through the hard times and struggling to find my way back, I had developed my own very personal relationship with God.

I view the elderly quite differently now. I feel that perhaps society on the whole does not recognize their quiet, sometimes unnoticed contributions. I thought about another very special individual who had touched my life. Like Walter, he would never know how he had dramatically changed my direction in life and it all began with a simple deed. My Dad received a phone call one night from an elderly relative we had never heard of. His mother and my Dad's mother had been cousins. This wonderful man had been researching the family history and our branch of the family tree was a missing piece of his work. He had contacted the relatives in Ireland and they gave him my Dad's address. He found us.

I suppose we could have furnished him with some family details for his book, and that would have been the end of that. But something inside of me told me, that this call was much more important. My Dad thought about it for awhile, and told me he had remembered his own mother talking about this man's mother and other members of that side of the family many years ago. Some of the family emigrated and some did not. They had all lost touch over the years and the family drifted apart.

I was curious, and for years had regretted not asking my grandparents for details about my family when I had the chance. When they died, it just seemed to be something I could only wonder about. I sent him a letter and explained where I fit into the family tree. In return, he sent me mountains of wonderful information, some of which I already knew but most of which I didn't. I sent him biographies of our family members, and he sent me detailed information of our enormous family and photos of my own great-grandfather. He sent me church records and cemetery maps with locations of interest and places with historical family significance in Kerry and Cork, just in case I wanted to see things for myself.

He sent me stories of the family history, descriptions of their homestead and tales, legends and events which took place as they were growing up. I sent him a photo, a surprise photo of his grandfather's old blacksmith forge building, which no longer exists. My Dad had taken the photo in 1960 on his first visit. He gave my Dad and myself the path for contact with our family in Ireland, and he opened the door for many wonderful unions, reunions and special friendships with our relatives who had emigrated to the United States in the 1950's.

He gave me something wonderful. He gave me my family. One year, on St. Patrick's Day, I opened my mailbox and found an amazing gift from him. It was the best gift I had ever received in my whole life. It came at just the right time in my life and it was priceless. He sent me microfiche which contained transcribed church records from Ireland with data that went back hundreds of years. He recognized my deep desire to connect with my past, and knew that it was important that I began my own journey.

That simple phone call he made one night changed my life. He was now eighty, and like Walter, showed me how a single individual, regardless of what age or stage of life they were in, still had the power to touch other people and help them along their own personal journeys. What an extraordinary gift to give to someone whom you had never even met. I hope to do the same someday for someone else.

The really important things left to do on my list, are the simple things. Simple, but all very important in their own way. There are eighty-seven of them in all left on my list and I have a lot of work to do. I also feel like I will be having some fun and plenty of adventures along the way too. I smile as I read them. Some of these things will be easy and others will take some courage. There was a time when I thought I might become a volunteer at Dad's facility. Most homes rely to some extent on volunteers to help with many kinds of activities and special events. I would be good at that. I have not forgotten my promise to join the ranks of those Meals-On-Wheels Angels either. Someday, just not right now. It is too soon. Everything has its time. To everything there is a season, a time for every purpose under heaven.

# XXXIV

## Walter's Lessons

Prior to his illness, Walter had given me some very good advice throughout the years. He was a wise man, and was very selective and sensitive about giving advice, but whenever he did, I always listened. If he had been aware of all of the events which had taken place since his illness, he would have been saddened to know that his journey affected our lives the way it did. He would have been saddened to see how this had affected me, or rather how I had allowed this to affect me. He can no longer speak for himself, but if he could, he would have told me several important things.

Walter would have told me that if I was ever faced with a life-changing hardship, to understand and accept my own limitations. Simply put, to just do my best. Walter would have told me to take care of myself. He would have suggested that I read the "Care Giver's Burnout List" first, and would have told me not to be afraid to seek help early if I was in trouble. He would have advised me to not make something a life's mission if things were beyond my control and were becoming self-destructive.

Walter would tell me to accept things for what they were. He would tell me that emotional turmoil would hold me back from living my own life. He would tell me to always keep my sense of humor and to be happy. He would remind me that one can't always control life's events or others' behavior, one can only control their own behavior. He would remind me that we are human, and it's far too easy to get caught up in judging others, wasting valuable energy trying to work out what is "fair." He would tell me that all things in life happen as they should. In the end, he would smile and tell me I did a good job. He would have thanked me. He would tell me that he loved me.

My fear had always been that the events of this journey and my way of handling each event would change who I was. I was always fighting that, as I liked who I was. When I was younger, I had always been able to scratch my way back whenever I became lost as I traveled along, but this time was different. This time I was afraid of the person I would become. I guess I had never experienced such an emotional upheaval which lasted for so long, for so many years. I lived in fear of making mistakes which would affect someone I held so dear.

Like all good backseat drivers, it became clear that I held a false perception of being in control. Like all good backseat drivers, I could make an abundance of noise, but truth be told, I was never in control. I was never in control of anything. I struggled with wondering who was actually driving whom. Was I really in that car at all? Maybe I was still standing on the pavement, scratching my head and looking around as the big black Buick of life pulled away from the curb without me so many years ago. No . . . now that I think about it, we spent an awful lot of time driving around in the back seat of that big black Buick. That was the place, you see, where Walter taught us so many of our valuable lessons.

We had some amazing discussions as we traveled along in the back seat of that car over the years. We talked about family. Dad often recounted stories of his parents and grandparents, growing up in town, his days in the Navy, and his romance with Mom which lasted more than fifty years. He talked about David, Ray and Jackie, and stories of their childhoods. He talked about their vacations and his work. We often drove to his job sites. He was always very proud of the blasting jobs which he was a part of, including one of his last jobs, the ledge blasting which was required for the building of the nursing home which was to be his last home. It was in the back of that faithful black Buick, that we all rode silently behind the hearse as we accompanied Mom, when she made her final journey to her resting place.

It was a place which brought us on many adventures, to very happy and exciting events, and to very sad events. Most of the time, they were just uneventful events. We always enjoyed just going for a drive just to look at the leaves in the fall, the twinkling lights in the winter, the flowers in the spring, and maybe just out for a "creamer" in the summer. It was an important place, because whether the destination was good or bad, whether we were happy or sad, we were always traveling as a family.

Some friends of the family have told me that they never went to see Walter once we took him from his home because they wanted to remember him the way he was before his illness. I can respect that. Every person has a right to deal with things in their own way. I didn't always understand, but now I can respect that. At times, that's how I felt too. It is a difficult thing to watch someone you love slipping away. It is painful. I guess I could have stepped back early on in the journey but I couldn't, and I wouldn't. Something told me to see it through until the end, and I will never regret that I did. Not only will I not regret that I did, I am proud of myself for doing so. I heard a voice from above. He said . . . "You go girl!"

I did make mistakes when it came to caring for Walter, but because my intentions were always good, the mistakes went unnoticed. In fact, they now seem irrelevant. But all of those experiences were an important gift. It took years for me to see that. It was only through living those life's experiences, could I understand and appreciate how Walter had helped me to find the genuine good in a bad situation. He helped me to grow and he helped me to find my way. It seems to me that when life hands you a challenge and things are really at their worst, that's when you discover just who you really are. As I look back now, I can see that I have changed. I am different now, and I like the person I have become.

# XXXV

# Waiting for God

The notice came in the mail. I always felt a slight pain of anxiety upon opening the mail box and finding a letter from Dad's facility. I momentarily paused before opening it as I sensed trouble. It's been a while since there was trouble, so maybe it will be okay. I let out a tiny sigh of relief. The festive announcement of the annual winter ball requested the honor of our presence. It was a formal type of affair, and we were again requested to deliver Dad's best suit for the occasion. I made my way to the closet, where Dad's cleaned and pressed suit carefully hung, still in the plastic dry cleaning bag. His crisp white shirt and his one remaining favorite tie were also ready and waiting. His polished shoes and a lone pair of socks sat quietly on the shelf. There was very little I had left of Dad's belongings, but I guarded his suit with care. It was one little thing I could still do for him well.

The day approached and we received a call from the facility, reminding us to deliver his suit in advance so they would be able to have him dressed and ready for the ball. We did as requested and pulled out our own best attire. David and I both had to work that day, so we decided to bring our clothes with us and change at work so we wouldn't have to go home first. I looked at my camera and video camera bags, less than enthusiastically, while trying to decide if I really wanted to save the memories this year. David had visited Dad yesterday, and said that Walter seemed to respond to his voice with a glimmer of recognition, and so we decided to bring the cameras.

I arrived at David's shop after work that day, all gussied up and adjusting my attitude for the festivities. David was quickly dressing, trying desperately to tie his own tie. Three attempts later and it was perfect. David looked handsome, and so much like his Dad. With everything tucked in and in place, we were on our way. I was excited to be seeing Ray and his wife, but David said they had called that day and said they were both sick and could not come.

We arrived a little late. Friday night traffic was unusually heavy, and the parking lot was full at the facility. At last, we found a spot. We sprang from our vehicle and sprinted to the door, out of breath as we quickly typed in the security code. We could hear the music already. Ahhhhh . . . The familiar sounds of Glenn Miller playing "String of Pearls." We made our way through the crowd, looking for Walter. Where was Walter? No Walter. After several trips around the facility, we made our way to Walter's room.

Dad's room was dark and he was in bed. His suit hung in his closet, his polished shoes on his dresser. No one had bothered to get him ready. He was forgotten. I felt that pain in the back of my neck again and I was angry. Do I once again open my big mouth and complain or do I quietly grind my teeth some more? This story is much bigger than the story of Dad. This is a story of elderly neglect. I didn't quite know what to do. Was there a roof top high enough where I could shout all of my complaints about society in general?

Dad wasn't asleep, he was just lying there waiting. David and I quickly got him out of bed and ready. Dad was confused, seemingly unaware of who we were and why we were undressing him, and putting him into these unfamiliar clothes. Dad looked different. He had lost more weight, and his face seemed to have changed. I didn't remember him looking so drawn before. I looked at the sores on his arms. He was so frail, just standing there in his "Daddy diapers." Once again, his prescription socks were nowhere to be found. He was cold and shivering as the two of us worked in haste to get him ready.

Could this suit really be his? Did I make a mistake? This shirt and suit were just too big, and seemed to hang from his tired frame. His shoes didn't fit either as his legs and feet were painfully swollen. We had no choice but to put on his old Velcro close sneakers. We combed his hair and I pinned a single white rose on his lapel. We slowly made our way toward the music and found seats in the community room.

Photos of last year's event were displayed on the wall. As the music played, I made my way to the wall of photos. There we were. Dad looked much different then. He was smiling and his eyes twinkled. His suit fit nicely. Dad was in the middle, with a smiling and twinkling David on one side, and me on the other. Yes . . . a smiling, twinkling little family photo. There were also photos of my old friends who were no longer with us. I smiled just a bit as I remembered how they touched me. I won't forget them. I won't forget how they changed me.

I sat back down and looked around the room. There were so many strangers. Sad faces, dressed up in fancy clothes and propped up in chairs. The chairs were aligned in tidy rows. I could immediately spot the new family members with that look in all of their faces, I knew it well. They all had those wide-eye expressions with smiles on their faces and cameras in their hands. They wore hopeful, yet strained expressions. They were all very attentive to their own loved one, putting great effort into coaxing their lost mother or father into responding to the festivities. That was me once upon a time, but not this time. Dad sat expressionless, slumping and looking at the floor.

The music did not seem to reach him this time. I reached out my hand and asked Dad if he wanted to dance. He did not understand my words. David encouraged him and he slowly rose. I led him to the dance floor and made myself smile. I remembered how he loved to dance, but not this time. I remembered how he would hum and sing, but not this time. The music ended and I slowly guided him back to his chair. His eyes shifted back to the floor.

A woman in her eighties was seated next to him. She wore a fancy yet rumpled peach-colored gown and sported a blond curly perm. Someone had obviously gotten carried away putting her make-up on. I did not know this new face. She was touching a man seated on the other side of her. He kept pulling away and eventually rose and left. She then turned her attentions toward Walter. At first she just rested her head on Dad's shoulder. When Dad did not respond, she began touching him and grabbing at his hand. Dad pulled away and his face looked angry.

She was not going to give up easily. In a flash, she again grabbed his hand and held on tight. She was pulling at his clothes with her other hand, her wrist corsage hitting Dad in the face. Her daughter was watching, smiling and amused I guess, a newcomer with her camera in tow, probably thinking it was sweet. The daughter moved in for a better shot. There it was . . . the flash of the camera. Dad was confused and not happy. Just who was this yellow-haired hussy playing fast and loose with Dad anyway? Dad started to get up. The woman started to topple over and the daughter flew into action to retrieve her mother, shooting an evil glance at Dad.

David and I grabbed Walter and led him back to his room. He had had enough and wanted to go to bed. We undressed him and began the search for his pajamas. While David took him to the bathroom, I pulled two more blankets from his closet and made his bed. We tucked Dad in and I bent down to kiss him goodnight. I carefully retrieved his suit of clothes. Tomorrow I would wash and press his shirt, iron his tie and reassemble his suit in the garment bag. I would wash and fold his socks, polish his shoes and carefully put it all back in that sacred section of my closet, where it would wait . . . for the next event. It was a long quiet ride home, and we silently climbed into our own pajamas. David plugged his tape of the dance into the VCR. He had captured only a few minutes of the event on film before putting his camera away. Dad's face was distant and expressionless. Walter was tired.

A week or so had passed when David popped in for a visit. It was mid-morning when he arrived at the facility. He found Walter asleep in his bed. It didn't matter what the time of day, we could always find Walter in bed. The room smelled bad. David spotted several puddles on the floor. Dad's urine was dark, very dark in color. Somewhat startled at the unwelcome sight, David began his search for the nurse. She summoned a maintenance person to clean up the mess, but was not too awfully alarmed at the dark urine. Walter stirred a bit, but couldn't really focus on David. Dad quietly repeated that he was cold. David reached out and touched his arm. He was cold to the touch. They kept this place very warm at all times but even dressed and under layers of blankets, Walter was cold. David rummaged through Dad's closet to find him another sweatshirt.

The dark urine was something I had read about, back in the days when I had that need to know everything about everything. Sleeping most of the time and being cold were also signs which were familiar to me. Walter now had little interest in life, the world or the people around him. He was separating himself somehow from his life here. Whether he knew it or not, or whether he had control of it or not was not important. It was happening. Things were progressing with that text-book accuracy, progressing it seemed, a little faster than I had sadly anticipated but nonetheless, it was happening and I was prepared. I could still do one last thing well. I could hold Dad's hand.

There was a time in my life which I felt I would somehow fail Walter unless I was frantically moving mountains for him. I now know, without question, that I did not fail Dad, as I was here today and simply holding his hand. It was all so simple, yct I ncvcr would have learned that one very important lesson in life if not for Walter. I smiled at him as he slept. He would never know how he changed my life. He would never know how much I loved him for teaching me so many things I needed to learn. All of my self-discovery happened because of his struggle with Alzheimer's, and in turn, his lovely tapestry touching me and enriching my own as well.

A person from the facility contacted us later that week. My lovely calming acceptance, and peaceful state of mind seems to be shattered when the phone rings. It seems that they had recently noticed that Dad was losing more weight. (Recently???? . . . Hello . . . Was he dehydrating as well? Were his kidneys slowly shutting down? One does not have to be too awfully brilliant to know that very dark urine was a bad thing.) We were told that Dad was not eating, and had been having increased difficulty when attempting to eat regular meals.

They needed our permission to start him on a regimen of high-nutrition liquid shakes. Do some families actually say no to this, or what? Are some residents just observed as they slowly starve? I guess they needed our permission as there was an additional cost for such care. What about the families who could not afford the additional care? What about this . . . what about that . . . ? Yes, we would greatly appreciate it if you people would attempt to give Walter his high-nutrition liquid meal. Thanks for calling.

It was Sunday morning. I opened my eyes to see Patrick sitting patiently at the foot of the bed, staring at me with those large emerald eyes. This could mean only one thing. The bowl must be empty. This was a refreshing change from the usual paw in the face at 4:30 A.M. I rolled over to look at the clock and was surprised to see that it was almost seven o'clock. I had a troubled night of sleep, and appreciated Patrick's newly acquired yet uncharacteristic patience. David was sleeping peacefully. He never really talked much about losing his mother, and I hoped that he is okay with where we now are with Walter. He and his Dad were so close his whole life, and he was very much like Walter. Like Walter, David is a good man, and a very caring human being, also a man of few words.

I listened to him breathe as he slept. It seemed a lifetime ago, during those very dark days that I simply wanted to leave. My mind was made up at that time, and that was that. It really wasn't so long ago come to think of it, yet now everything was different. I guess when I really thought about what I first loved and admired about him years ago, I came to realize that all of those feelings were still alive and well these twenty-five years later. We have been through a lot together and I couldn't even bring myself to imagine my life without him. He was my best friend. I would be there for him, and he was going to need me. As David and I traveled along that sometimes bumpy road, one thing was clear. We were both in that car together. One of us may have been doing the steering, but the other was always holding the map. At times we would argue, debating which direction we would go. Each role was different. Both roles were equally important if we were going to find our way.

David's life would be different one day with both of his parents gone. David had mentioned once, only once, that he wondered if Alzheimer's had any genetic link. He was bothered by that. I knew what was on his mind but I couldn't respond. Who knows what each of us has in store as we journey along our personal path. The future would take care of itself somehow. I am living for today. With that thought in mind, I quietly slipped out of bed as Patrick's newfound patience was wearing thin.

I made myself a pot of coffee and turned on the news. It seems that studies show that one needs to drink juice. Studies show that there is a link between the antioxidants found in fruits and vegetables, and the effect on Alzheimer's statistics. Studies show that three servings of fruit or vegetable juice per week could reduce the occurrence of Alzheimer's by 76%. I roll my eyes as I wonder just who was compiling the data on that study. Walter drank his morning juice every day of his life. Do you mean to tell me that after years of mind-boggling in-depth research by the experts, this was the answer? Just where did they come up with this 76% anyway? Those pharmaceutical companies making their millions on "life enhancing" drugs will be distressed to hear this.

I see that there is an envelope from Dad's facility sitting on the counter. It arrived several days ago and has been neglected. It sits unopened. I wonder what jolly affair they are cooking up next and I open it. It is a calendar of events for the following month which would knock one's socks off. Each day is jammed full of events comprised of games, trivia, culinary classes, music, entertainment, creative arts, puppet entertainment, scarf dancing, afternoon tea and sing-a-longs. There will be poetry, Mexican hat dancing, senior jokes, spelling bees, who's got the button, down memory lane and stretch-n-sing. I see that there is a rigorous evening program scheduled for each day on the calendar. God bless the events coordinator. She has got her hands full. I recall sitting in on many of these types of events. It is not an easy job being the cheerleader for a room full of people who are lost, silent, unresponsive or confused.

It was not really all that long ago that we prodded a reluctant Dad out of bed just to get him outside for a short walk. We chatted up each flower of the lovely landscape just for something to say. What was interesting to me was that Dad could not distinguish color any more. David stopped at a bed of Black-Eyed Susans and proceeded to point out to Walter the yellow-orange petals and brown centered blooms, but Dad could not repeat back what was told to him. David and Dad moved to the next bed where identical clusters stood. Dad just stood there, shaking his head, not able to recall the colors. We moved to a patch of green shrubbery. David held a leaf in his hand and gave it to Walter. Dad studied it, turning it over and over again, thinking for a long time before saying he did not know what color it was.

How I wish I could walk in that man's shoes for just ten minutes. Was he not seeing color anymore? Was he seeing it but not comprehending the meaning of color? Was he seeing it all clearly but the thought process just abruptly stopped?

Did he just forget the question? Was the world really in black and white and it is our own imagination which perceives the colors we are seeing? What is the meaning of life? If a tree falls and there is no one around to hear it, does it make a noise? Does that little light in the refrigerator really go off when you shut the door???? Here I go again. Some things just are as they are. I can not be Walter for ten minutes, and God willing, I will never have to know what it is like to walk in his shoes.

I found myself saying "Dad doesn't know us anymore" to anyone who asked, just to sum it all up in a nutshell without a lot of further explanation. What was interesting to me was that he didn't recognize himself either. He looks in the mirror and seems confused as to just who is looking back at him. David brought in photos of a recent event held at the facility. He showed Walter a nice photo of the two of them together. Walter did not know himself. He did not know who David was either from the photo. He appeared surprised when David pointed out the man in the photo was Walter himself, and the man next to him was his son.

David asked him if he knew his son's name. Dad said he didn't know. David told Walter that he was his son, and Walter thought that over for a little while before he said, "You're a nice boy." David drew a long exhausted breath and explained to Walter that he, Walter was his father. David said, "You are my Dad . . . .and you are the greatest Dad in the whole world." David leaned over and kissed his father right in the middle of his forehead as he spoke. Walter responded without hesitation, "Thanks Dave." Dad then immediately shot David an astonished look. "Where did I get that?" Dad said. "I know your name!" He had even surprised himself.

I was dumbfounded, not that he got his name right or that somewhere in there on some hidden second level he still knew us. I stood in awe as I had known these two men for twenty five years and had never heard something like "You are the greatest Dad in the whole world." He kissed his father! Did he just actually kiss his father? Yep . . . I saw it! David had finally learned that it was okay to express a sentiment like that out loud to his Dad. I was so incredibly proud of him. I was so glad he said it, and I knew that someday soon, he would be glad that after fifty-four years, he finally told his Dad the way he felt about him for all of those many years. There would be no looking back with regrets after Dad was gone about things that were never said. This was a huge lesson learned. You need to tell people you love, just how much they mean to you while they are with you, and not wait for enough courage to say it later with regret after they are gone.

Walter came up with David's name, and that was incredible. It made me think. It was a message of hope to those of us everywhere who feel lost or abandoned ourselves when the aging parent viewed their children, family and friends as strangers. Those memories of loved ones may appear to be long gone, but I prefer to believe that they are all intact, safely tucked away. The recall ability may be hindered by these tangles of ganglion, but those memories and feelings are still there. It is a blessing and joy when an inadvertent tiny piece fights its way through these road blocks as a small reminder that our determination to love, and their ability to breakthrough to those they love can not be stopped by this disease.

I recalled years earlier, when the comment was made that "Dad was just an empty shell of a man." I ground my teeth and stuck to my belief that this was wrong. That comment was the easy answer, or maybe an excuse to give up and look the other way. I am confident that the experts will come up with a way to dissolve this plaque formation which builds these barriers in the brain. They will conquer the disease someday. I look forward to reading the amazing testimonials of distraught family members who had given up hope, but because of medical advancements were able to be reunited with a once lost soul, the parent they loved so much.

I am confident that with these barriers gone, the memories will find their way to the surface again. We shall be amazed to discover that we, the children, were not merely faded memories gone or erased. We are memories blocked, struggling to find their way just as Walter proved to us that day. This man never stopped teaching us some very important things.

The hard part is watching the months roll by into years. I do not think a reunion of which I spoke will come in time for Dad, but I am happy for the families who may never have to witness the torment once a cure is found. Nonetheless, today would be a good day to visit Walter. I guess I once again needed to see for myself, just where everything stands before we gently update the rest of the family of his progression through the third and final stage. I had learned an important lesson about unresolved issues. They can be carried around like heavy baggage for many years, and they can be very destructive. I'm sure that there is not a soul alive who could possibly have any unresolved issues with Walter, but I still feel the need to give friends and family members the opportunity for a last visit, or a last broken bit of conversation, maybe a smile or glint of recognition from a faded memory of years ago.

Something like that could be very important to someone who cares for Walter as the years go by. It's interesting to me how the smallest of seemingly insignificant events are the ones we sometimes draw on years later. They say talking is good, and I'm sure it breaks through the barriers of Alzheimer's at some point even in the very final stages. I am content to just sit quietly and hold his hand. No longer am I driven to scrape up bits of idle chatter, desperate to keep the conversation rolling in the presence of Walter, just because silence can sometimes be uncomfortable. I am no longer compelled to test him. Talking was important then, not so long ago. It was so important to communicate our sense of caring to Walter in any form possible.

I made an observation recently that family, friends and even staff, not to mention myself all seem to gravitate to an interesting natural instinct or phenomenon when attempting to communicate with the residents at this facility. When the person you are talking to doesn't seem to understand you anymore, you simply raise your voice an octave, and shout louder. One forgets that their loved one is not deaf and this will not help them to understand. Most likely it is irritating. Why have I not realized it before? There is a lot of shouting that goes on here. I have this sudden urge to cross-stitch a plaque for the entrance area here which reads "Please Don't Shout At Your Loved One . . . They Can Hear You!"

I know what you're thinking. This type of place primarily cares for elderly residents and their hearing could very well be impaired. This is not always the case. I smile a bit as I recall communicating with Mom's caregiver from Armenia. She spoke English very well, but at times there were small language barriers. I am sure that there were times when I responded by kicking the volume up a notch in an effort to be understood. For some reason, that never worked. Silence is nice. Maybe Walter prefers the quiet now. Maybe our voices translate into a jumbled mayhem of noise inside his head. I don't know. For me, silence is better. Silence provides for necessary reflection.

I have been doing some reflecting lately and have found comfort with my understanding of the journey, which according to my map, draws to a close. I am ready for what comes next. I have a very small list of things which need attention, things which still bother me. Actually the list has only one item . . . Mom and her wish. The anniversary of her death approaches, and I always felt she was denied her death bed wish. She wanted that pink heart-shaped stone. Dad stated he did not want to spend eternity under such a thing, and the large plain grey stone they ordered after her death was adequate. Case closed.

Say what you will, but my job here is not over until it's done. It has been years now since that November day which Anne left us and only now have I hatched a plan which will help me sleep a little better. I wished I had thought of it years ago, but better late than never. It is really quite simple. I got out of bed this morning and pulled out a large sheet of paper. I drew a very simple heart with over-all dimensions of about fourteen inches. I loaded my font program on the computer and found a beautiful Edwardian script which I thought was gracefully appropriate.

I typed in a simple yet elegant "Mom" centered in the heart design. I tried "Mother" and quickly back spaced it out and retyped "Mom." She was "Mom" to her children, and even Walter called her "Mom" throughout the years. I will have a heart-shaped foot stone created in lovely pink granite using the script engraving. It will be installed flush to the ground at the foot of her plot and will go seemingly unnoticed to a casual passer-by. I will know it is there. Anne will know it is there. Her wish fulfilled, and Walter can be at peace knowing it's not on his side. Perhaps it is not about simply filling someone's wish. Maybe it is my own personal way of telling Anne I loved her. It's too bad I didn't say it to her when I had the chance.

I will remain steadfast, unwavering in purpose and loyalty in my agreement with Anne to see Walter through until the end. I don't have a lot of answers as to the why's and how's but I do know this—A wise woman once said, that each journey with a loved one with Alzheimer's Disease is unique. This is true. A wise man once said that when a person is diagnosed with Alzheimer's Disease, it affects not only that individual, but also affects all those who love them. This is true. The book said, "Read the Care Givers Burnout List

early on and do not be afraid to seek help." Talk to people . . . talk to people . . . talk to people. Simply finding out
that you are not alone is the greatest comfort of all.

I am here to say to anyone touched by this, that you
too, will experience a painful and life altering experience in
helping a loved one through the three stages of the disease,
using whatever methods you need to keep them safe. You
will discover and develop your own unique problem solving
abilities as you encounter each unexpected challenge. You
will have good days and very bad days as conditions deteriorate. You will develop a special gift which will enable you to
reach out to a friend, neighbor or even a stranger when they
muster the courage to share the grim news that their loved
one is experiencing the all-too-familiar first signs of Alzheimer's. You have the ability to reach out and help a person
like "Maggie" simply by sharing.

Those who persevere will find they have the amazing
ability to help others with their life's tapestry as they create
their own. Those who persevere through to the end will also
experience a wonderful silver lining. They too will discover
as I did, that some answers would never be found. Some will
discover that all they need to know is very close to home. It
is a long personal journey for all involved. Often, it is a story
which begins with the person afflicted with Alzheimer's, but
ultimately is the story of the close circle of individuals who
have surrounded that person with love, understanding and
care. In an often desperate mission to help the one they
love, they would begin their quest in search of answers, years
and many miles later, only to find . . . themselves.

Walter's room was dark. We arrived to find him in a
deep sleep on top of his covers. The room had a bad smell,
but at least there were no puddles on the floor this time.
We tried to gently wake him but he was too far away. We

decided to let him sleep, when David made a discovery. Walter's now baggy pants were on backwards, zipped and buttoned with his belt tightly buckled in the back. We indignantly made our way to the nurse's station. This was the last straw. Up until now it was the battle of the missing socks and shoes on the wrong feet. How could they possibly not notice they were putting his pants on backwards? Our huffy emotional tirade was interrupted by a calm and rational explanation. He was dressed that way intentionally. The staff could not keep up with the constant bathroom problem behavior, and even with the Daddy Diapers, they simply could not always be one step ahead of him. They dressed him that way so he would have no choice but to go in his diapers. We were abruptly silent. We suddenly understood the gravity, the finality, the loss of that last shred of dignity.

We returned quietly to Dad's room and again gently tried to wake him. This time he stirred and opened his eyes. He looked up at us and softly said, "I was almost dead."

David said, "Dad, you must have been having a good deep sleep."

Dad responded in full sentences, "No . . . I was almost dead, and it was very nice there." He proceeded to tell us that he was near "the light." His facial expression became concerned as he warned us that you couldn't get too close, otherwise it would be too hard to get back. He repeated that it was very nice there. I was shocked, but this was Walter, and Walter never lied. I asked him if he saw any people there and he said he had. I asked him if he saw his parents there. He thought for a moment but he wasn't sure. I pointed to a framed picture of Anne and asked him if he saw Mom. He thought for a moment but he wasn't sure. I don't recall exactly what was running through my mind just then, but for some reason I asked him if he heard any music. He said no, he didn't think so, but again repeated that it was very nice there.

Whatever Walter had experienced, be it real or imagined, he was peacefully content. He described his experience in sentences. I wondered how after all of those months of broken thought patterns, he was able to communicate so clearly. It was nice to hear his voice again. We understood without really understanding. I left that day with a feeling of bewilderment, a strange indescribable excitement of sorts and an overwhelming sense of peace. I was going to be fine with whatever happened next, because Walter was fine with it. The world is full of believers and nonbelievers, yet none of that mattered. His words, "It was very nice there," warmed me from the inside out, and I will never forget his last message of hope for all of us. That was his final gift to me. Walter truly was a kind and gentle soul.

The call came quietly in the wee hours of the night. I did not cry. Promise Number Three was now completed. Although Walter became too far away for me to reach, and I could not back seat drive him all the way to the end of his journey, it has been my extreme honor and privilege that he allowed me to come along for the ride for as long as he could.